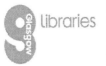
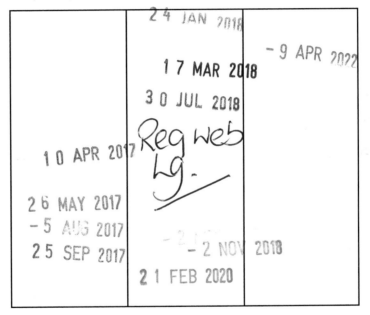

How to Cook Healthily

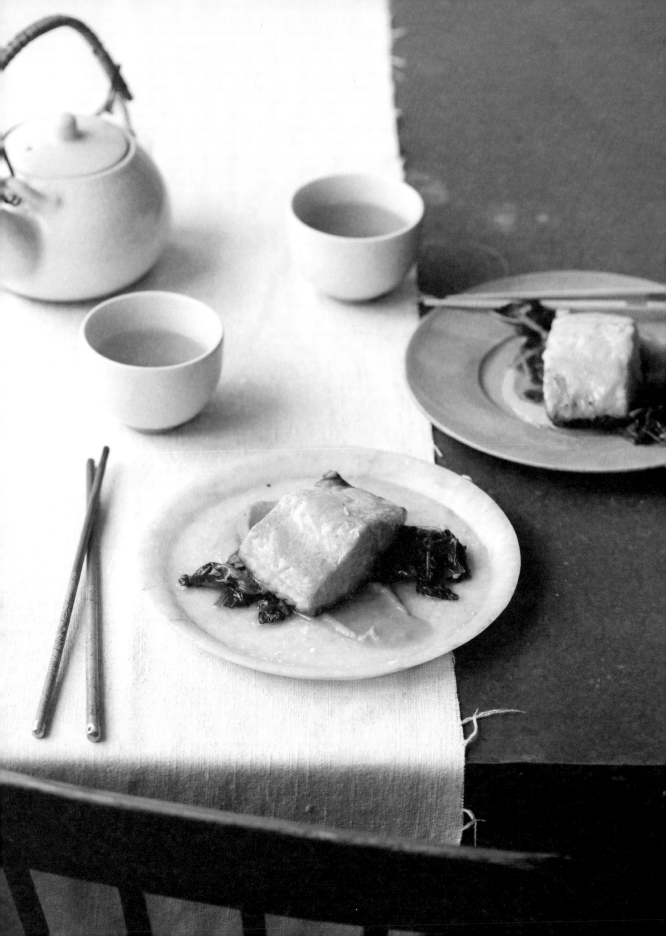

How to Cook Healthily

Dale Pinnock

**Simple techniques and
everyday recipes for
a healthy, happy life**

Photography by Issy Croker

The
MEDICINAL
CHEF

quadrille

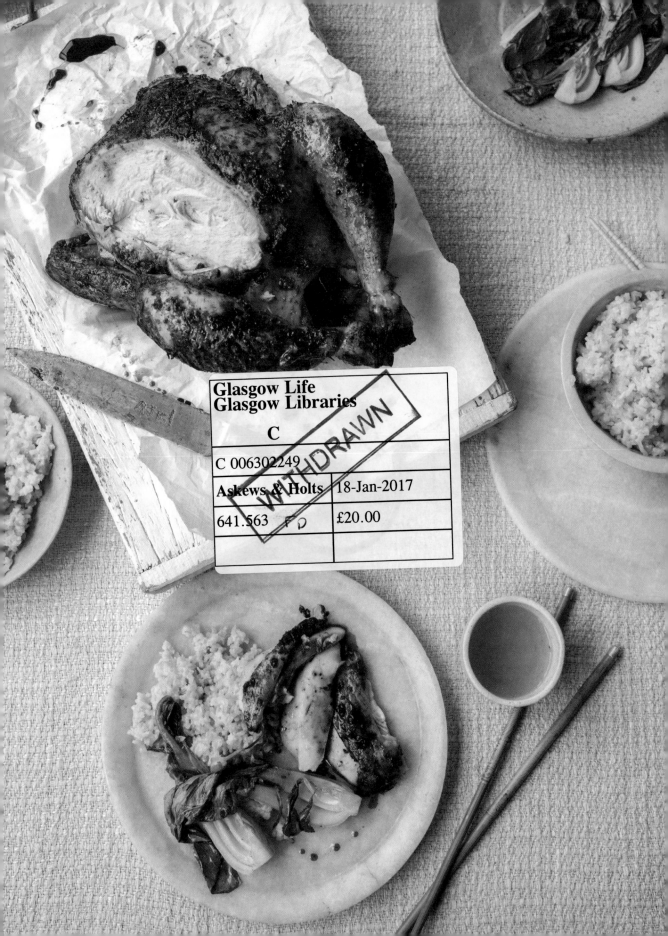

Contents

Introduction

In recent years it has become blatantly obvious that the food we eat affects our health in a massive way. We are seeing first-hand the extent to which bad diet can influence the health of nations. Globally we are seeing levels of degenerative disease and mortality rates that are just staggering. These aren't deaths from things like infectious disease, war or genocide... these are deaths in their hundreds of thousands from things that are for the most part completely avoidable. Type 2 diabetes, for example, affects 415 million people, and by 2040 it is believed that it will affect one person in ten: that's 642 million people. This isn't the congenital condition type 1 diabetes that we develop in childhood: this is a condition that comes from lifestyle. I'm not throwing around blame, but it is what it is. In the UK we have 160,000 deaths a year from cardiovascular disease.

And as for cancer statistics, we all know where these are going: currently they state that one in three of us will be directly affected by cancer in some way during our lifetime, and those odds are getting worse. What we are seeing here are the terrible consequences of intervention in our diet: refined rubbish sold to us in the name of convenience. We are constantly reminded how time-poor we are (although if we really analyze our days, we may be surprised how much time we do have). We are being sold this processed rubbish under the guise – and this is what I find incredibly sinister – of a "healthy option". And we use cartoons and sporting heroes to sell it to our children. We get addicted to the high levels of salt, sugar and trans fats. Many food giants exploit our increased financial strain and churn out cheap processed produce, positioning themselves as heroes who are there to save us money and help us put good food on the table. The whole thing has gone horribly wrong and we seriously need to go back to basics. But... what ARE these basics? Where do we start? Well, this book

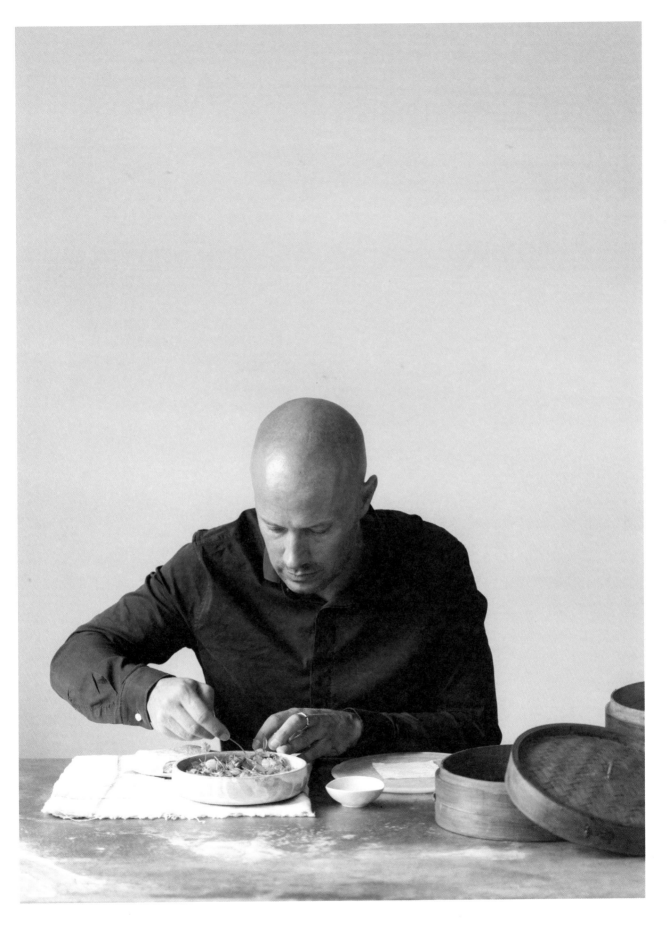

will help to give you some support there, and there are two little mantras that will tell you everything you need to know. Firstly: "If it ran, it swam, or it grew… then eat it!! Everything else, leave out." This basically tells us to get back to whole ingredients that are found in their natural original state, as nature provides them. A brightly coloured box with an ingredients list as long as *War and Peace* and that sounds like the contents of a chemistry set is NOT a natural state. The second little mantra is even simpler: "Real food does not contain ingredients. Real food IS ingredients."

So, why did I write this book? Of all the questions I get asked and of all the advice that people often want, the basics of where to start and how to start putting a healthy diet together are always at the top. I think almost all of us want to eat more healthily. The problem is that we are constantly bombarded with all kinds of weird and wonderful information. New diets, fads and strange ingredients abound. Which is it this week: the Himalayan wonga wonga berry, or biodynamic grass-fed unicorn? To many people, eating healthily seems out of reach. It may be that we think it's complicated, or expensive. We may just think it is plain boring or, like so many, we just don't have a clue where to start. Let's face it, it isn't

really taught in our schools. Sure, we may have cookery classes, we may learn about protein, fats, carbohydrates etc., but when do we ever get taught the basics of putting a good diet together? What should be included? What types of fats should I use for cooking? What cooking methods are the best? What on earth am I supposed to do with quinoa? Over the past few years I have looked around the book stores and have seen several celebrity chef "How to Cook" type books. Then it dawned on me: there really should be something like this about cooking healthily. So I decided to put one together, and here it is.

The purpose of this book is really to be a guide for you to help you make sense of what healthy dishes look like, how they are composed, and what cooking methods you can use to create a healthy dish and to get the best out of your ingredients. It will give you some key information as to what is beneficial in certain ingredients. Ideas for side dishes, main courses, healthy salads, sweet treats: it's all there. There is a bit of everything. I don't necessarily want this book to be 100 per cent instructional. Don't see this as being your entire healthy repertoire. I want this to be inspiration for the way in which you cook for life.

WHAT IS COVERED:

COOKING TECHNIQUES

I have dedicated a few chapters to some of the best cooking techniques for preparing healthy food and getting the best out of fresh ingredients. Here you will find wonderful stir-fries, recipes to make in your steamer, and hearty oven-baked dishes.

HEALTHY INGREDIENTS

Other chapters focus on some of the staple ingredients that make up a healthy diet. You'll find sumptuous salads, gorgeous fish and seafood dishes, ideas for meat and poultry, and ways to bring whole grains to life. These chapters aim to show you not only what is good about these ingredients, but also the diverse ways in which these ingredients can be used.

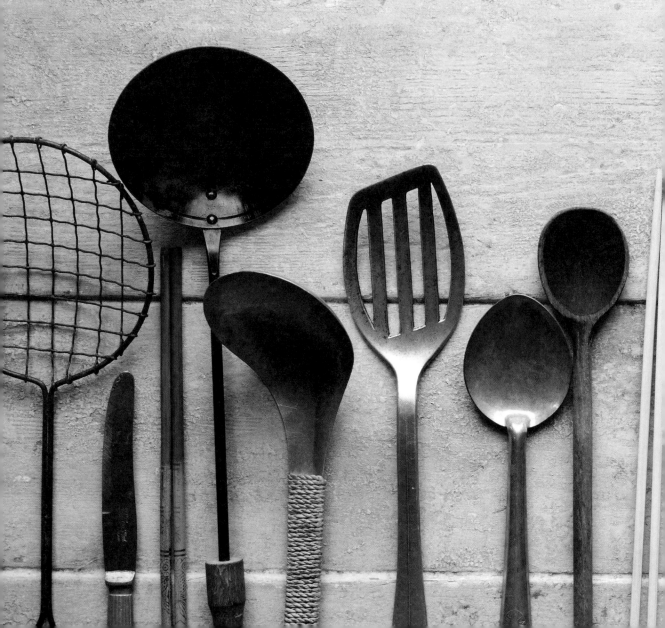

PART 1:
Techniques and Ingredients

Adopting healthier cooking methods couldn't be simpler. For me, there are only really two rules you need to follow to make a huge difference.

The first, and the one that is probably obvious by now, is to go easy on the deep frying. This is mostly an exercise in reducing your intake of refined vegetable oils. For the most part, things are deep fried in the likes of sunflower oil. This is extremely high in something called omega-6 fatty acids (which will be covered later in the Good Fats section) which, when consumed in anything more than tiny quantities, can trigger inflammatory damage to areas like the cardiovascular system. These oils are also very prone to oxidative damage, so after one or two uses the oil becomes a soup of damaging free radicals. Certainly in commercial establishments, the oils used in fryers are not changed after each use.

The second rule for healthier cooking is to avoid cooking your vegetables to death. Who remembers Sunday lunches when the broccoli was almost transparent, and the greens started to turn grey because everything had been boiled for half the day? Not only does this create an utterly unpleasant meal, but boiling vegetables for too long destroys almost all of the important nutrients – many of which are water soluble and heat sensitive.

So, with the above in mind, you will see that healthier cooking really isn't restrictive at all, and you have a lot of methods left in your armoury to create a huge range of dishes. Let's take a quick overview.

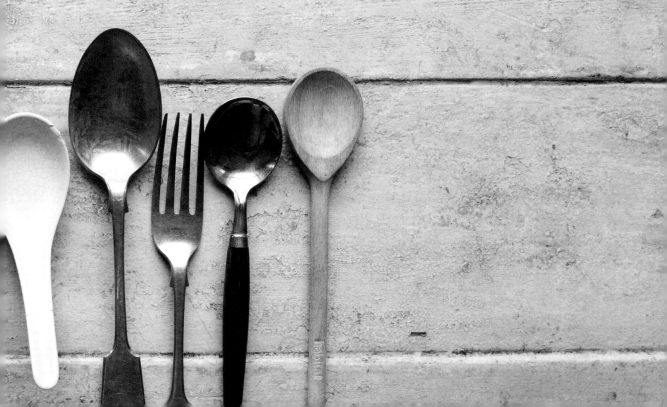

Roasting and Baking

Roasting and baking make the preparation of healthy ingredients an absolute joy, in my opinion. It is a perfect method for combining all manner of flavours and textures, and turning simple healthy staples like root vegetables into some of the most comforting and sustaining food imaginable.

This method of cooking is especially good for the winter months. Just think of the abundance of casseroles, layered bakes and gooey, comforting foods – crispy, crunchy, earthy, wholesome loveliness. Such lovely food that often requires little attention once the basic prep has been done, so it's a great option when multitasking of an evening. Many of these types of dishes are great for family meals. They are rich, tasty, warming and, most importantly, incredibly nutritious. Healthy meals don't have to be all rabbit food and rice cakes!

RECIPES

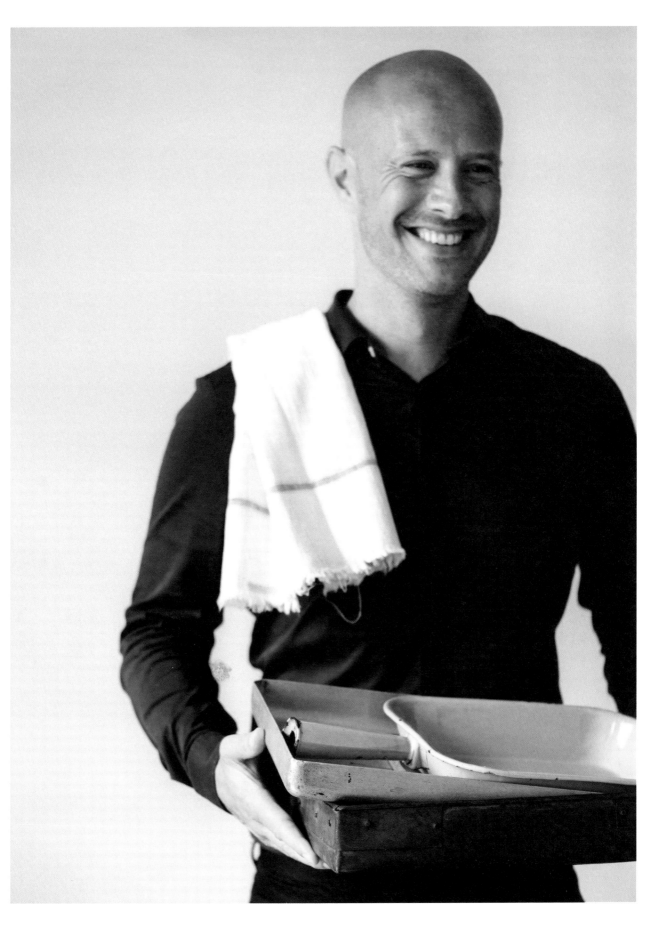

Steaming

Steaming was once a super-trendy way to move towards healthy eating. While it has dropped out of fashion a little bit, it remains one of the healthiest ways to cook that there is.

As a cooking technique, it preserves nutrients, doesn't require additional fat to be added, and is very quick. As I've mentioned before, many of the important nutrients found in vegetables are water soluble. The B vitamins and vitamin C, for example, can easily leach out when vegetables are boiled, so it can sometimes be the case that drinking the water the vegetables were cooked in may provide more nutritional value than the vegetables themselves! Steaming is one way around this, as it conserves a far greater proportion of the water-soluble nutrients. Just make sure you steam them until they are just softening, rather than all the way to a mushy consistency.

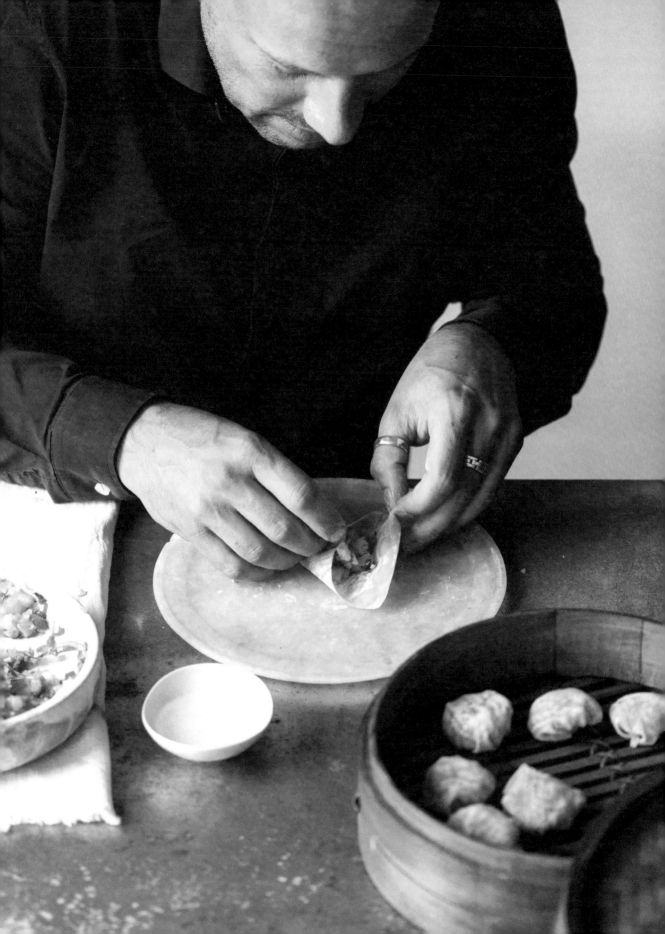

Stir-frying

Stir-frying is perfect for modern-day life, as it ticks two big boxes: speed and nutrition.

One of the biggest gripes I hear from people who want to start eating more healthily is that they lack time. If that is your concern, too, then stir-frying could be your saviour. The cooking is done on a high heat so that ingredients cook quickly. What's more, you can say goodbye to over-boiled grey, tasteless vegetables in which valuable, water-soluble nutrients such as vitamin C and the energy-giving B vitamins have dissipated. Stir-frying keeps things nutrient rich, crisp and fresh.

MY FAVOURITE STIR-FRY INGREDIENTS
This is just my top five!

CAVOLO NERO
Sometimes called black kale, it has good levels of magnesium, non-haem iron, antioxidants and fibre.

LEEKS
They add additional depth of flavour, cook quickly and are great for digestive health thanks to their prebiotic properties.

SHIITAKE MUSHROOMS
Good for immunity thanks to a special group of sugars they contain called polysaccharides that are known to influence cells such as natural killer cells in the immune system.

RED/ORANGE (BELL) PEPPERS
High in antioxidants, mostly in the form of carotenoids.

RED CABBAGE
Packed with flavonoids, hailed for their cardiovascular-health benefits.

RECIPES

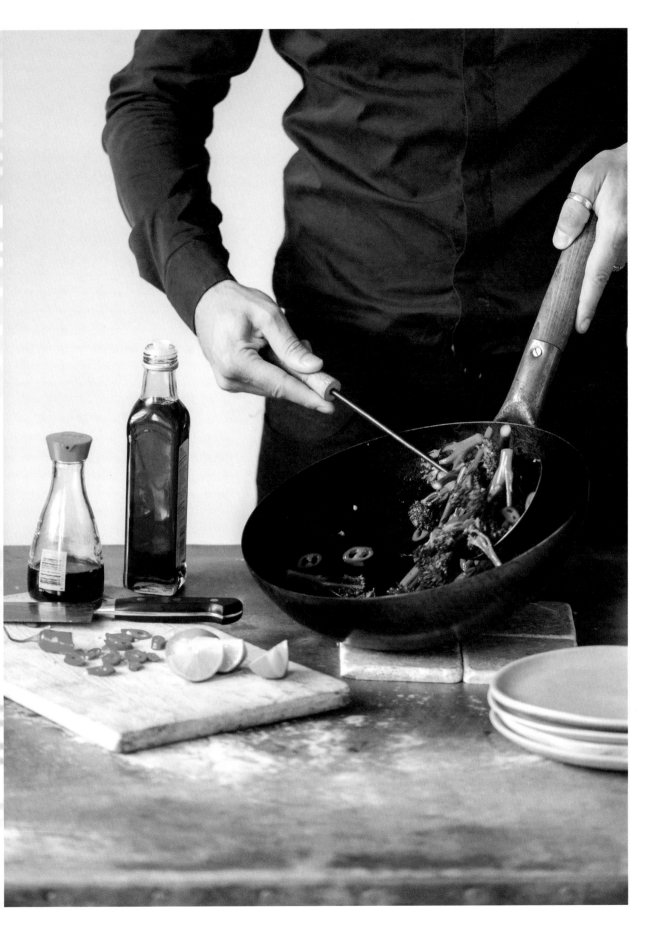

Good Fats

We have a strange relationship with fat in the UK and USA. We either avoid all fats like the plague and opt for low-fat diet rubbish, or we indulge in gallons of the wrong types of fat.

For decades we have been fed the message that fat is the enemy and will kill us faster than anything. We have been encouraged to cut out fat at every opportunity, and also to swap around the fats that we use – avoiding the saturated and increasing our intake of the supposedly "good" or "heart-healthy" vegetable oils. This recommendation represents one of the biggest public health disasters of all time – more on that later. Fats are a vital group of nutrients, essential for virtually every aspect of our health.

We just need the right types of fats, and the benefits will be enormous, especially for the heart, joints, immune system and mental and emotional health.

WHAT IS GOOD AND WHAT IS BAD?

This is one area that has been the subject of great debate in recent years, and advances in research and data analysis have revealed that the recommendations we have been given for decades have been horribly wrong. These recommendations caused us to change the types of fats and oils that we use, and as a result have altered our intake of vital substances called essential fatty acids that have significant effects on our health.

Essential fatty acids are a group of fats that are biologically active and critical for our health and the health of every single cell in the body. They are called "essential" because we have to get them from our diet; our bodies cannot manufacture them. There are two main classes of essential fatty acids: omega 3 and omega 6. You may have heard of omega 9, too, but the body can actually convert omega 6 into omega 9, so obtaining it is of far less concern. These fatty acids play such a vast and varied role in human physiology that it is really rather mind-blowing.

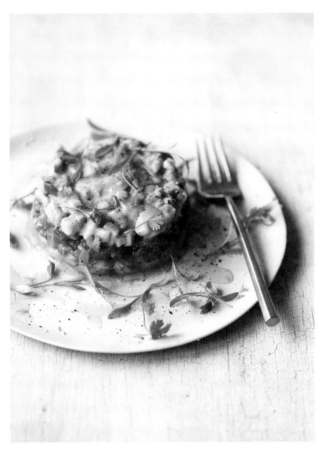

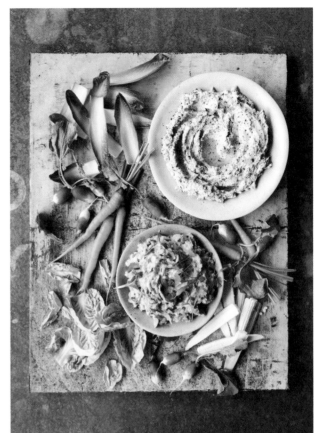

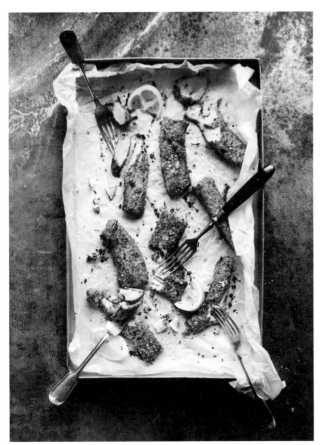

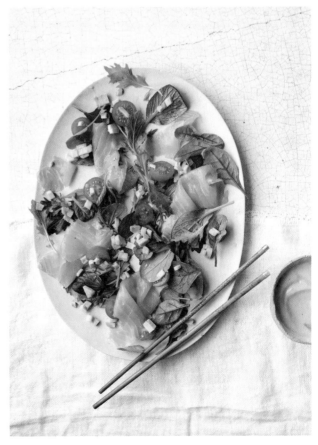

All great so far. However, our intake of these fatty acids cannot just be left to chance. We need to get some balance, and I strongly urge anyone reading this to become acutely aware of how to achieve omega balance (my previous book *The Power of Three* goes into great detail about this and shows you how to achieve this in the food that you eat.) So why do we need balance? If we consume too much of one fatty acid, then we can unleash a whole world of problems upon our physiology. The problematic one that I am talking about is omega 6. Omega-6 fatty acids are used for normal brain function, growth and development. However, we only need a VERY small amount of these per day in order for them to achieve their physiological goals. The good thing is that omega 6 is so ubiquitous in foods, you will only be deficient if you become a breatharian and stop eating!

When we consume both omega 3 and omega 6, they go through a series of metabolic pathways. These are streams of chemical reactions that alter them and transform them into end products that play various roles in our bodies. When we consume our required amount of omega 6, it is converted into several important substances that do their jobs nice and quietly. The problem arises, however, when we consume too much omega

6, which then gets shuttled down a slightly different metabolic pathway and begins to form something called a "Series 2 prostaglandin". This active compound actually switches on and exacerbates inflammation. Here is the final lightning bolt: in the UK we are consuming – PER DAY – on average 23 TIMES more omega 6 than we need. This means that the average person following a typical British diet will be putting themselves in a state of chronic (i.e. ongoing, long-term) sub-clinical (i.e. not immediately obvious and only revealed by blood tests) inflammation within tissues.

Why is this a problem? Well, low-grade chronic inflammation is linked to many of the chronic diseases that plague us in the West. Heart disease, for example, is essentially caused by inflammation. Inflammation of the endothelium (the inner skin of blood vessels) is the first thing that occurs. The body then responds to this and attempts to repair it, and this is when substances like cholesterol get caught up in it and plaques begin to form in the arteries. Inflammation of the endothelium also makes the vessels less responsive to natural variations in blood flow, contributing to elevated blood pressure.

Chronic low-grade inflammation is also an important factor in the aetiology of cancer. Ongoing inflammation in a tissue can activate certain genes and affect the natural cycle of cell replication. So being in this state is serious, but you won't be aware of it, as it is a slow burner that gives no signs.

So, how on earth did we get into this mess in the first place? Thanks to the public health recommendations I mentioned earlier. It was from the mid 1970s onwards that the message about our eating habits and what constituted a healthy diet started to change drastically. Massive public-health campaigns persuaded us that saturated fat was the devil and was the thing in our diet that would ensure an early grave. We were encouraged to opt for "heart healthy" vegetable oils and margarines and we were all cooking with sunflower oil and slathering margarine on our toast. Food manufacturers, wanting to appear like the good Samaritans, heeded these campaigns too, and started using "healthy" vegetable oil in their foods. And there we have it. Suddenly our intake of vegetable oils was way beyond anything that would have ever occurred in our natural diet. Bang: the fatty acid balance took a nosedive.

OTHER HEALTHY FATS

OLEIC ACID
This fatty acid is found in abundance in olive oil, and is believed to be one of the factors that make the Mediterranean diet so healthy. It is an omega-9 fatty acid that is known to reduce LDL cholesterol.

MEDIUM-CHAIN TRIGLYCERIDES
(MCTS) are found in oils like coconut oil. They are a type of saturated fat that displays very different behaviour than many saturated fats from animal sources. They require little or no digestive intervention, and pretty much go straight into circulation to be used as a convenient energy source. There are all manner of claims made about these oils, such as their ability to enhance "fat burning" and physical performance. I would take these claims with a pinch of salt, however, as the evidence so far isn't particularly strong.

WHY TAKE IN PLENTY OF GOOD FATS?
A regular intake of good fats can have an amazing impact on heart health. They can lower cholesterol, reduce systemic inflammation and reduce blood pressure. They can help with inflammatory conditions. They help to maintain a healthy brain and nervous system, too.

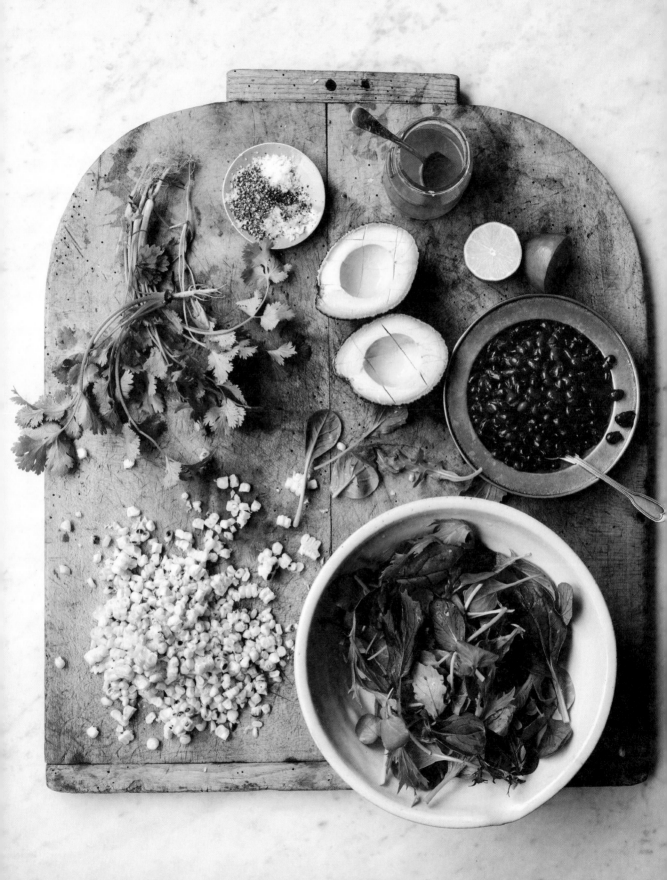

TOP FOODS FOR HEALTHY FAT INTAKE

I try to encourage people to get some good fats into each meal. Not only does this ensure you get a good spectrum of them into your diet, but they also help to fill you up as they slow gastric emptying and influence "satiety" hormones.

If you can, buy eggs that are fortified with omega-3 fatty acids. Drop sunflower and "vegetable oil" and switch to olive oil and coconut oil for your cooking. Drizzle olive oil onto your salads or cooked vegetables.

OILY FISH
Salmon, mackerel, herrings, tuna, sardines: these are the richest sources of omega-3 fatty acids on the planet, and the omega-3 fatty acids they contain are preformed, which basically means they can be used by the body straightaway.
Top tip: Swap bacon or ham in a sandwich for some smoked salmon.

AVOCADOS
A great source of oleic acid and GLA.
Top tip: Try adding some sliced avocado to your cooked breakfast in the morning.

SEEDS
Rich in GLA, vitamin E and the plant form of omega 3 – ALA. Whilst ALA isn't useful as an omega-3 source per se, it does reduce the metabolism of excess omega 6, so has a role to play.

COCONUT OIL
A rich source of medium-chain triglycerides.
Top tip: Coconut oil is especially good for Southeast Asian and Indian cooking.

RECIPES

Mixed seed houmous: **page 49**

The best-ever guacamole: **page 50**

Avocado and smoked salmon salad: **page 68**

Tuna carpaccio with orange dressing: **page 149**

Feel-good fish fingers: **page 150**

Whole Grains

Whole grains are an absolute staple ingredient in a healthy diet, for very good reason. Many of you may know that I am not a huge advocate of eating large amounts of carbohydrates, and would always advise that we ditch refined carbohydrates for a lifetime. But adding some key whole grains into your diet can certainly offer some real benefit.

Whole grains are often rich in a vast array of vitamins and minerals, have a high fibre content, are a great slow-release energy source, and deliver some interesting health benefits. Among the reported health benefits, there are a few that have been researched extensively, and that we have great understanding of, so it is let's explore these a little further here.

DIGESTIVE HEALTH
One of the greatest woes that the modern Western diet brings with it is a rather broad cross-section of digestive maladies. Bloating, gas, cramping, IBS, constipation... the list seems endless. Some of these are directly related to diet, and others can be managed partly by diet. The modern diet that many of us follow in the West is sadly heavily laden with processed convenience foods – ready meals and pre-packaged foods.

White bread, white rice, white pasta: these all play havoc with digestive health. One of the main reasons for this is the lack of fibre in processed foods. Fibre is vital for digestive health for two main reasons. First, it physically works as a bulking agent. It bulks out digestive content and in doing so it helps with digestive transit. Fibre absorbs water, several times its own weight in water, in fact, and when it does this it swells up. This makes the stool enlarge and begin to stretch the walls of the digestive tract. Within the walls of the gut are stretch receptors. Once they detect the stretching that swelling fibre instigates, they then stimulate the rhythmical contraction of the gut known as peristalsis. This undulating contraction is what allows the contents of the gut to move through and be removed with ease.

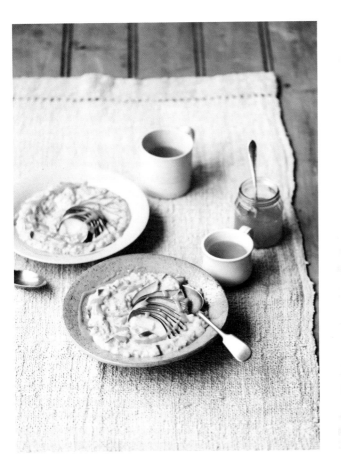

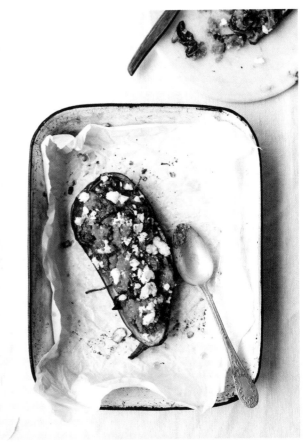

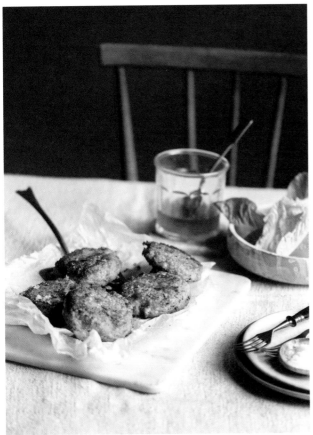

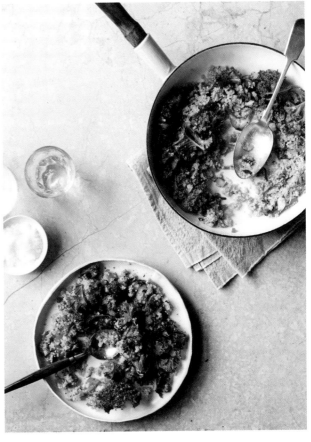

The second way in which fibre benefits digestive health is by influencing gut flora. "Gut flora" refers to the colony of bacteria that live in our digestive tract – not problematic bacteria, but actually a friendly, beneficial army that is 100-trillion strong! Dietary fibre can help to keep this massive colony healthy. Some of the more dense and complex fibres will actually get fermented and broken down by the gut flora, and when the bacteria ferment these compounds, two things happen: they actually cause the bacteria to multiply and increase in number, and the bacteria can release by-products during the fermentation of this fibre. These by-products include compounds like butyric acid, which actually instigates repair mechanisms within the large intestine, helping to keep it healthy.

CARDIOVASCULAR HEALTH

Whole grains have a very long-standing reputation as a food that benefits cardiovascular health, and have been the subject of many trials in this context. So, how exactly could a whole grain benefit the health of the heart? Well, it comes down to their impact on cholesterol. Whole grains can lower it, by a rather interesting

mechanism all to do with the soluble fibre that is found within them. Our body produces cholesterol naturally; it is a vital and necessary substance. We produce it every single day in the liver. When it is produced, a very large percentage of it is indeed actually used in digestion. It is used to make bile acids, which are substances released from the gall bladder that help to break down fat globules into smaller particles that can be more easily absorbed in the digestive tract. When the bile acids have done their job, the cholesterol within is then liberated and absorbed further down in the digestive tract, where it enters circulation. This is an ongoing loop.

Now, the soluble fibre in whole grains, particularly fibres such as the beta-glucan found in oats, actually forms a gel-like substance in the digestive tract. This substance will bind to cholesterol that has been recycled from bile acids and prevent it from being absorbed as it normally would. Because there is less cholesterol being re-absorbed, and because it plays such an important part in the manufacture of bile acids, the body will mobilize cholesterol that is in circulation for use in bile acid formation. The end result is that our blood cholesterol levels go down.

GLYCAEMIC RESPONSE

As I have stated many times, I don't necessarily advise people to eat large amounts of carbohydrates – think of them as an accompaniment rather than as the base of a dish. As well as reducing carbohydrate portion sizes, the type of carbohydrates that we consume are the real key. This is why whole grains are the best choice. Because they are so high in fibre, they take much longer to digest than their white, refined alter-egos (think brown rice over white). This is of vital importance to our long-term health, due to the impact that this has on blood sugar.

White refined carbohydrates contain virtually no fibre at all. This means that they take very little digestive effort and are digested rapidly. Because of this rapid digestion, they can release their glucose content into the blood stream quickly, which floods and overwhelms it. In the long term, consuming high levels of refined carbohydrates that flood blood sugar can cause a significant number of health issues, from Type-2 diabetes to contributing to cardiovascular disease. (This is covered in greater depth in my book *The Power of Three*.)

Whole grains, on the other hand, are digested much more slowly due to their fibre content, and as a result they drip feed the blood sugar. This places very little burden on the insulin system, and bypasses many of the problems that come with flooding blood sugar and over-taxing the insulin system.

There are now huge amounts of whole grains commercially available, with more and more coming to market all the time. However, I have a few favourites that I feel are the absolute best of the bunch, that have been well researched and documented, and are great staples of all manner of international cuisines.

BROWN RICE

This was one of the original health food staples from long ago. It always conjured up images of vegetarian restaurants and old health-food stores. How times have changed. Now it is everywhere and so widely used. From a nutritional point of view, it is, in my opinion, one of the best.

KEY NUTRIENTS:
B vitamins: energy production, regulating nerve function, stress
Manganese: helps with the formation of connective tissue, clotting factors, and the metabolism of protein and carbohydrates
Selenium: supports thyroid and immune functions, helps produce the body's own in-built antioxidants

Gamma-oryzanol: an antioxidant that helps lower cholesterol
Fibre: helps increase digestive transit and lower cholesterol

HOW TO PREPARE:
I like to rinse rice a few times before covering with water and simmering for about 20–25 minutes.

BULGUR WHEAT
Bulgur wheat is that wonderful grain that forms the base of the classic tabbouleh. Slightly sweet, and nutty, it is one of my absolute go-to ingredients.

KEY NUTRIENTS:
B vitamins: heart health, energy production, nerve function
Betaine: lowers homocysteine
Very high fibre: satiety, blood sugar management, improved digestive transit, reduces cholesterol

MILLET
This wonderful grain is slightly less common, but you can buy it in any health-food store. It has a lovely nutty flavour, and is in fact very versatile – it can even be made into a mash. I have included millet here as it has a very broad nutritional profile.

KEY NUTRIENTS:
Copper: helps make red blood cells, supports immune and neurological health, involved in collagen formation

Phosphorous: the second most abundant mineral in the body; involved in maintaining bones and teeth
Magnesium: involved in more than 1,000 chemical reactions in the body daily, as well as in regulating muscle function and supporting neurological health

HOW TO PREPARE:
This is a super-easy grain to prepare. Cook it for about 15 minutes at a constant simmer.

OATS
Oats are one of the real staples. I am appalled at the array of hideous breakfast cereals that are marketed as being some kind of healthy option for us, especially the rubbish marketed to children. Oats really do come to the rescue. When they are not covered in sugar and overly processed, oats are a fantastic, nutrient-rich, slow-release energy source, so for those of you who like a cereal at breakfast time, oats are the number-one choice.

KEY NUTRIENTS:
B vitamins: convert food into energy and support a healthy nervous system
Beta-glucan: soluble fibre that has been clinically proven to lower cholesterol
Manganese: formation of connective tissue and clotting factors

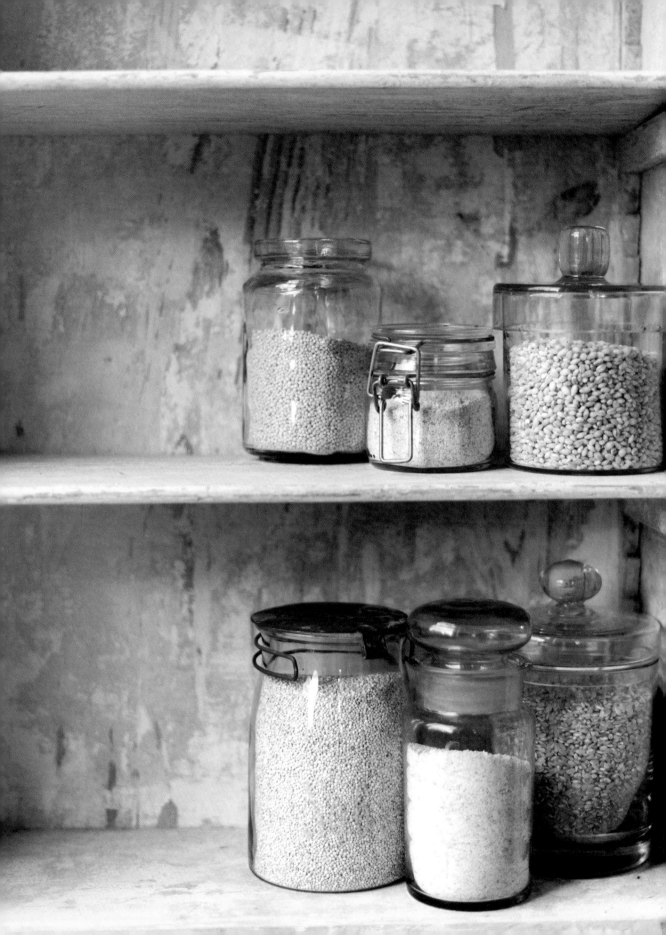

Avenathramide: cardio-protective antioxidant

HOW TO PREPARE:
I generally do about 1½ –2:1 ratio of liquid to oats when making porridge. Oats are also fantastic for baking and for topping dishes, and they cook very quickly.

PEARL BARLEY
Pearl barley is another one of my favourite grains. I use it as an alternative to rice when I make risotto. As a grain, it is a super-slow burner compared to white risotto rice, and has a delicious nutty flavour. It is great cold in a salad, too.

KEY NUTRIENTS:
Molybdenum: involved in everything from energy production to stimulating our body to produce its own inherent antioxidant substances, looking after our cells
Chromium: a trace mineral involved in the production of Glucose Tolerance Factor, for regulating blood sugar levels
Also B vitamins and magnesium: (see above and page 28)

HOW TO PREPARE:
This is a tougher grain than others and takes a lot longer to cook for this reason. I personally prefer to soak it for about an hour beforehand to give it a bit of a head start before simmering for about 40 minutes.

You could even soak it overnight/all day if you wanted a shorter cooking time, of 20 minutes or so.

QUINOA
Quinoa, which used to be a strange, mystical ingredient that nobody could pronounce, has become massively popular in recent years; it is literally everywhere. You'll find it in ready meals, food-to-go outlets and every supermarket. This is one "trendy" food that I believe really does live up to its hype. For a grain, it has an extremely high protein content and high fibre content, which means that it takes much longer to digest than many grains, so it won't raise blood sugar levels rapidly. It is also exceptionally nutrient dense.

KEY NUTRIENTS:
Iron: carries oxygen to tissues
Zinc: involved in regulating white blood cell function, regulates sebaceous secretions
Folate: regulates cell division, involved in DNA production
Copper: collagen formation, immunological support, healthy nervous system, red blood cell manufacture

HOW TO PREPARE:
This is a super-easy grain to prepare and cooks in simmering water for 15–20 minutes. You know it is done when the grain enlarges, turns a clearer

colour, and a small tail-like projection forms on the outside.

The recipes here should give you a few ideas of how to use grains in diverse and delicious ways, whether it is whipping up a breakfast, making a tasty side, or using them as a base for other dishes, such as salads.

RECIPES

Salads

Salads are without doubt one of the main staples of a healthy diet. They can be the epitome of a healthy meal, but so many people fear the worst when they hear the word "salad". It conjures up images of droopy lettuce leaves and limp cucumber slices, like the salads of old, or the lifeless heap that used to be served as a garnish. But please don't fear: that is not what I am talking about here. Salads are a way of bringing together as many minimally processed plant foods as possible, which is a vital part of building a healthy diet.

In this age, when so many of us are consuming large amounts of convenience foods, ready meals and processed food items, we struggle to get anywhere near the levels of micronutrients that we need on a daily basis. We certainly get the macronutrients (protein, fats, carbohydrates) from convenience foods (often way too much of them). But the micronutrients – the vitamins, minerals, trace elements and phytonutrients – are destroyed through heavy processing. If your diet is built around too many convenience foods, then chances are you won't be getting enough at all. I view a good, dense salad as almost a nutritional supplement. It is a meal that is guaranteed to give you a great injection of so many key nutrients, especially those that are damaged during processing and cooking, plus a great cocktail of phytonutrients – compounds in plants that aren't necessarily nutrients in the truest sense (in that you can't develop a physical condition from a deficiency in them) but that can very powerfully influence our physiology. So, with this in mind, I always try to make at least one meal a day a salad meal.

Before we get on to the recipes, let's take a look at the main nutrients that are damaged by processing: the B vitamins and vitamin C.

B VITAMINS

The B vitamins are some of the most commonly deficient nutrients in the western world. There are several reasons for this, but mostly it's that they are damaged very easily by heat, and are water soluble, so different

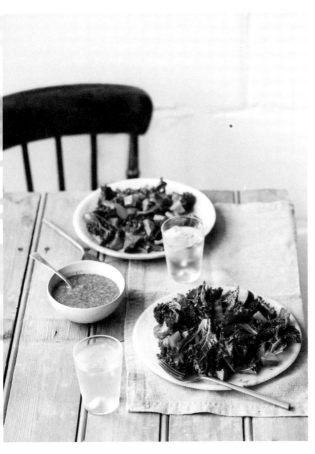

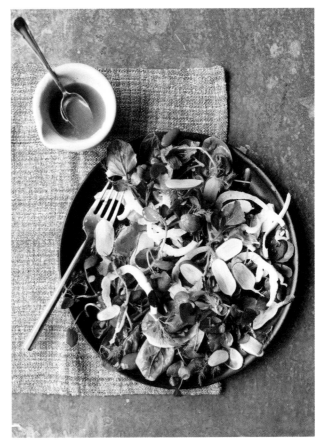

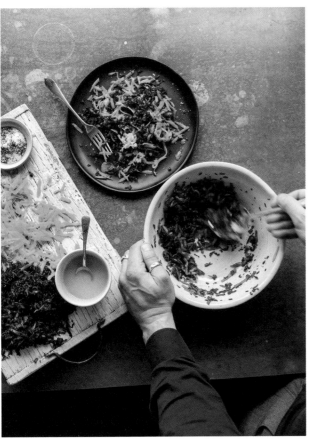

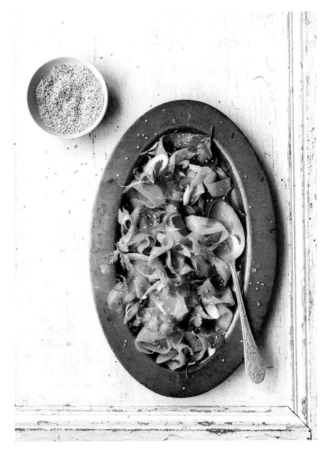

cooking methods can greatly affect the levels of the B vitamins in our food. B vitamins play very diverse roles in our body. Importantly, they are involved in converting food into energy at a cellular level. When glucose enters our cells, it needs to be converted into something called ATP, which is what the cells run on, and the B vitamins are vital for this process, and are also involved in making new cells in the body. Several of the B vitamins have a role to play in regulating the function of the nervous system and manufacturing neurotransmitters, and have been shown to protect the brain from premature shrinkage. Thankfully, these vitamins are found in quite a diverse range of foods, and it is just the way that we cook them that will determine whether they will stick around or not.

VITAMIN C

Vitamin C is probably the most famous of all the micronutrients, and the one that everyone thinks of when they start coming down with a cold or feeling under the weather. Vitamin C performs a considerable number of functions in the body. Firstly, as we all know, it is involved in immunity. Vitamin C is used by specialized types of blood cells to deliver what is called the "oxidative burst". This is a cloud of highly reactive free radicals that are released by this line of white blood cells when they come face to face with pathogens. This cloud of free radicals can kill susceptible pathogens. Vitamin C also helps with the motility of white blood cells, assisting in their migration to the site of infection, and is an important nutrient for the health of the skin. This is because it is involved in the production of collagen – a protein matrix that gives skin its structural integrity. A lack of vitamin C in your diet certainly won't help you to age well! It is important for the growth and repair of tissues, and is involved in making scar tissue.

MY FAVOURITE SALAD INGREDIENTS

As I have said, a good salad isn't about limp lettuce. It should be full of nutrient-dense vegetables. The list is endless but these are some of the ones I go back to again and again.

SPINACH

Spinach is one of the best leaves to use as a salad base. Instead of being mostly water with few nutrients, like most lettuce is, spinach is very nutrient dense. It is a great source of beta carotene, which is the plant source of vitamin A. This is important for the health of the skin and eyes, as well as being an antioxidant. Spinach contains quite high levels of vitamin C for its weight, is a great source of magnesium, and contains reasonable amounts of non-haem iron.

RED (BELL) PEPPERS

All peppers are a great addition to salads, but red ones are my favourite. These are packed with a group of compounds called flavonoids, which are part of the chemistry that gives peppers their distinctive colour. These compounds have been widely studied and are known to benefit cardiovascular health by widening the blood vessels and helping to lower blood pressure (as part of a healthy diet – a couple of peppers are no good to a chain-smoking, pizza-eating couch potato). They are also rich in beta carotene and have loads of vitamin C.

RED ONIONS

These are packed with those heart-healthy flavonoids that can keep blood vessels strong and help lower blood pressure. Red onions are also great for digestive health. This is because they contain something called inulin, a prebiotic – meaning that it acts as a food source for the bacterial colony that lives in our gut. The bacteria ferment inulin and break it down, and in doing so they grow and flourish. They also release by-products during the fermentation that help to repair and maintain the gut wall.

CELERY

Ok, so not the most glamorous of vegetables and definitely one of those love/hate type of ingredients, but celery is a little nutritional dynamo of sorts. It actually contains a massive array of antioxidant compounds, such as flavonoids, stilbenoids and phenolic acids. Celery also contains a class of compounds called phthalides, which have been shown to act as muscle relaxants, painkillers and also potent diuretics (as anyone who has drunk celery juice can attest to).

RADISHES

Radishes are one of those old-school salad ingredients that seem to have dropped out of fashion a little bit these days, but I think they are great, as they have some quite complex chemistry for such a simple ingredient. Firstly, they are rich in a group of compounds called glucosinolates. These compounds can actually increase the production of one of our own inbuilt antioxidant enzymes – glutathione peroxidase. This enzyme, aside from being an antioxidant, is also responsible for cellular "house keeping". Glucosinolates are known to be antimutagenic, too (meaning that help prevent the mutation of genetic material). Radishes also contain a great deal of flavonoids, which are beneficial for heart health and have antioxidant function.

WATERCRESS

Watercress has an amazing, robust, peppery flavour, and I love adding sprigs of it to a salad to give an

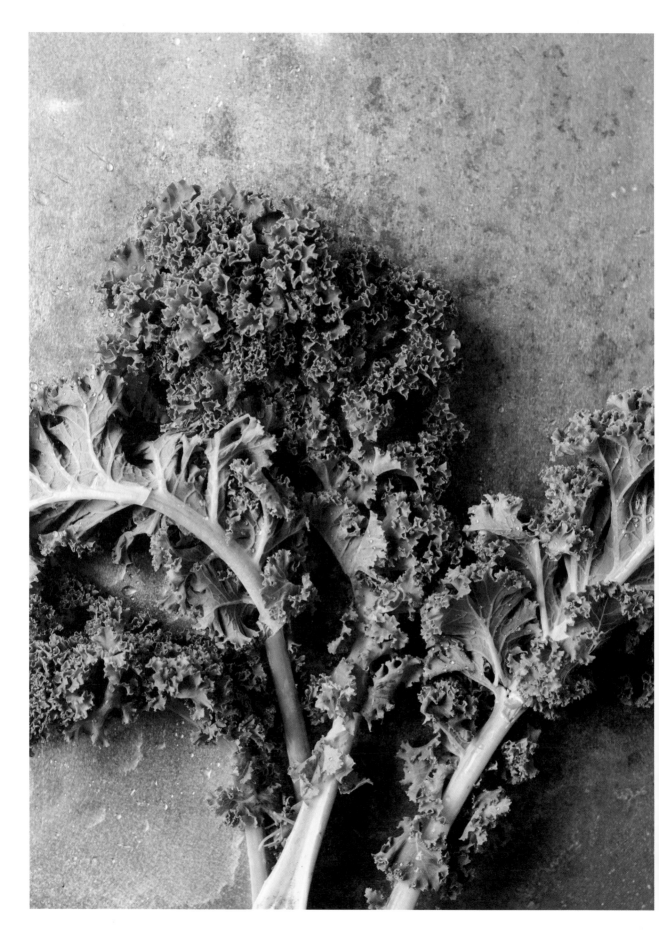

occasional heat hit. It is also rich in glucosinolates (see page 35). The most abundant nutrient in watercress, however, is vitamin K, vital for bone formation, protecting neurons and clotting. Additionally, watercress is very high in vitamin C – much higher than many fruits.

ROCKET (ARUGULA)

Rocket is another of my favourite salad greens, especially with a bit of goat cheese and some walnuts. A close relative to radishes, its chemistry is similar, with great levels of those potent glucosinolates (see page 35). Rocket is also rich in vitamin K, vitamin C and beta carotene.

KALE

This is certainly one of the trendiest ingredients around at the moment: if you believe what some people may tell you, kale should make you fly and walk on water. All of the hype aside, it is still a great ingredient, rich in vitamin K, beta carotene, vitamin C and non-haem iron. One thing that is particularly abundant in kale is the mineral magnesium. This commonly deficient mineral is vital for over 1,000 daily chemical reactions in the body. The magnesium in kale is found within the chlorophyll that gives it its deep green colour.

RECIPES

Meat and Poultry

There is definitely an assumption in the weird and wonderful world of health and nutrition that meat is super unhealthy. The number of glossy magazines, websites and forums that warn us to keep away from it at all costs is unbelievable.

While consuming it for three meals a day, seven days a week is definitely not going to do you any favours, it is still an important dietary inclusion. Now, if people decide not to eat meat from a moral point of view, then I could and would not argue against them, as it is a very clear and valid ethical stance. If, on the other hand, people avoid it in a quest to be healthier, that's a different story. Meat can give us a broad spectrum of vital minerals, such as haem iron, zinc and selenium. A few meat meals a week will give you vast amounts of nutrients packed into a small serving. You could view it as a flavoursome nutritional supplement in a healthy diet.

RECIPES

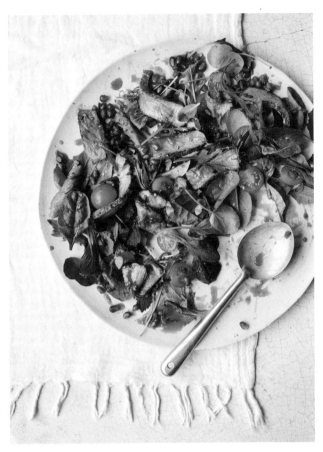
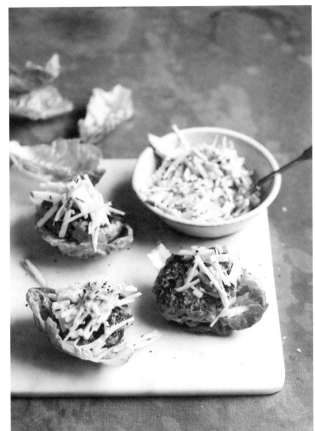
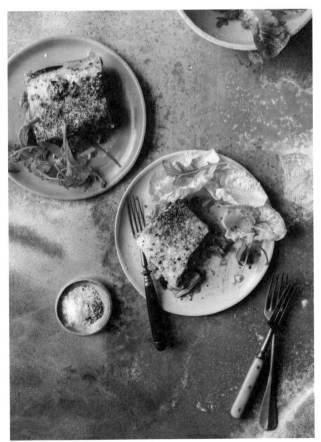
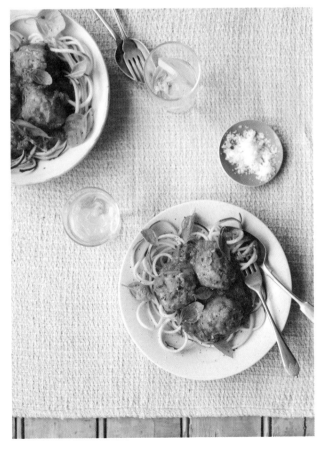

Fish and Seafood

Fish and seafood as a group of ingredients are so often overlooked in the diet here in the UK, which is a travesty: not only are they utterly delicious, but they contain some of the most important nutrients for our long-term health.

Seafoods such as shellfish, for example, are very rich sources of the mineral selenium, a nutrient that is seriously lacking in the West. This is due not only to a lack of consumption of seafood, but also to the fact that selenium in the soil is often depleted in modern intensive farming. Selenium is used by our body for several important functions. One of the main things that it does is help our body to manufacture its own inbuilt antioxidant enzyme family – glutathione peroxidase. This antioxidant compound helps to disarm free radicals in the body that can damage cells and trigger disease. Selenium is also important in regulating the function of the thyroid.

The second vital nutrient group found in fish in particular, especially the oily varieties such as salmon, tuna and mackerel etc., is omega-3 fatty acids. These fats are vital for almost every aspect of our health. Firstly they are anti-inflammatory. Fatty acids that come into our body from our diet are converted into compounds that regulate numerous chemical processes in the body. The most common group of communication compounds derived from fatty acids are called prostaglandins. These regulate, amongst other things, inflammation in the body. There are three types of prostaglandins: Series 1, Series 2 and Series 3. Series 1 and 3 are ANTI-inflammatory, and Series 2 switch ON inflammation in the body. Different dietary fats contain different fatty acids, and different fatty acids produce different prostaglandins. The omega-3 fatty acids found in oily fish, particularly one called EPA, produce the powerfully anti-inflammatory Series 3 prostaglandins. So why does any of this matter? Well, inflammation in the body is an important response in immunity and managing infection, but excessive inflammation can begin to damage tissues. We know, for example, that inflammation can damage the walls of our blood vessels. When this happens, circulating

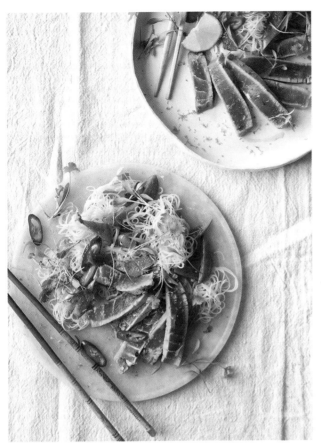
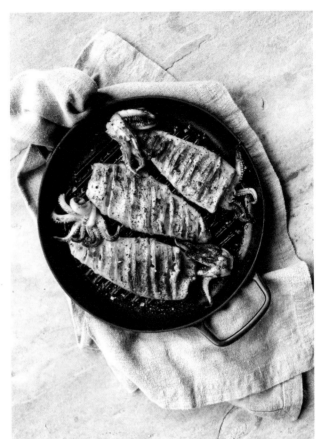
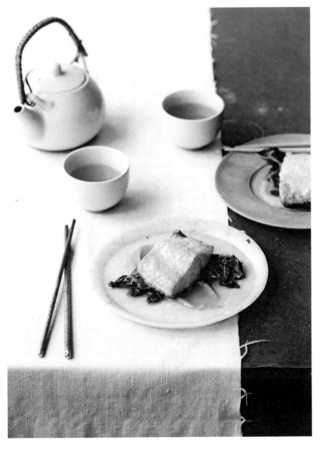
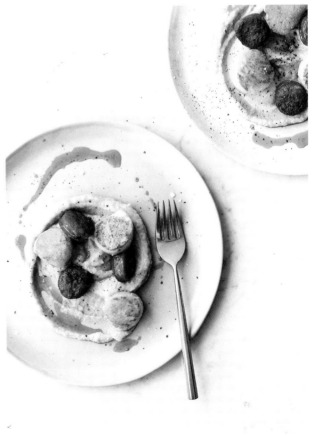

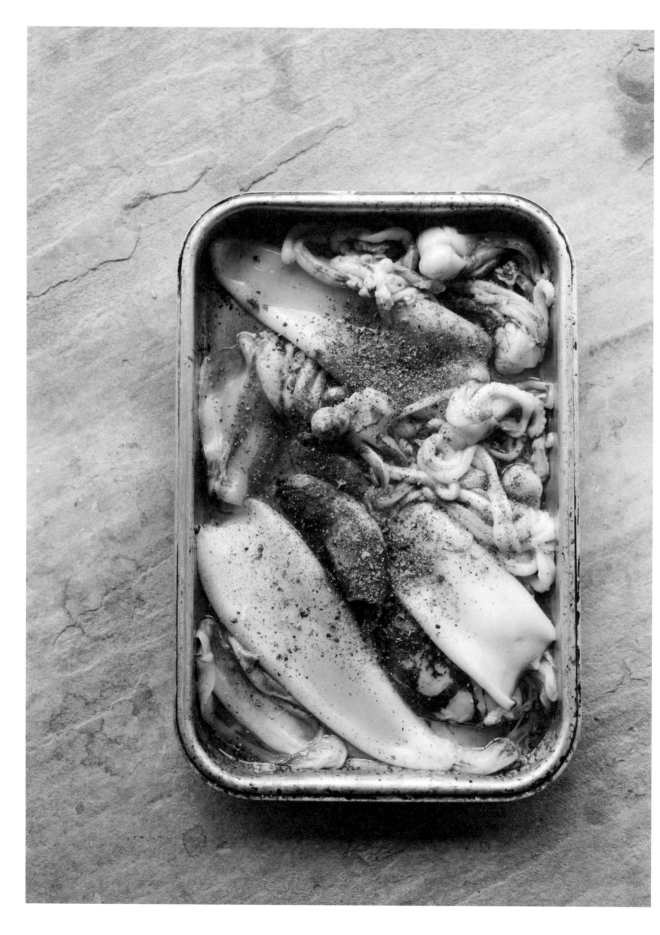

cholesterol can get embedded in the blood vessel walls, our immune system gets involved, and before we know it a plaque has formed which is an indicator of the early stages of heart disease. Long-term inflammation within tissues is also associated with many cancers, and inflammation can sometimes trigger certain genes that cause uncontrolled growth and replication of cells to switch on. So, managing inflammation is a vastly important part of looking after our long-term health and helping to prevent some of the most serious health problems we face in the modern world. Obviously, regulating inflammation can help with issues such as joint problems and injuries too.

Omega-3 fatty acids can also help to maintain the health of our brain and nervous system, can lower LDL cholesterol and contribute to healthy immunological health. Taking into account all of the above, I stand by my recommendation that increasing our intake of fish and seafood can be one of the most important dietary steps we can take towards greater health.

RECIPES

Sweets and Snacks

When we make the decision to start eating more healthily, very often we believe that we can no longer indulge our sweet tooth, and that we have to completely veer away from "guilty" snacking.

Well, this really doesn't need to be the case. Providing you make a few tweaks and changes, you can create some very healthy and nutritious snacks that you can always have on hand. And that's the key: being prepared and having healthier options available, so you aren't tempted to head over to the less healthy treats that you may be used to.

When it comes to sweet things, I'm not going to tell you that honey and dates, etc., are "natural sugar" and therefore acceptable to eat with abandon. Sugar is sugar as far as our insulin response is concerned. What these types of ingredients do offer that just a spoonful of sugar won't, is a few additional nutrients. This means that the calories aren't as "empty" – but please don't interpret this as a reason to guzzle them down!

There is one sugar substitute, however, that can be a good option when used correctly. This is stevia - a crystaline substance derived from a leaf. It is intensely sweet. The good news is that it has zero effect on blood sugar, as it isn't absorbed. Use it in much smaller quantities than you would sugar, as too much makes its flavour turn oddly bitter.

When it comes to sweet treats and desserts, it is very much possible to recreate many of your favourites, just by using different ingredients to achieve the same textures and flavours. This final chapter aims to show you that it's not all doom and gloom – healthy eating and indulgence can go together.

RECIPES

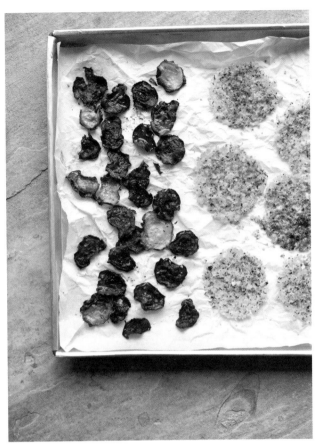

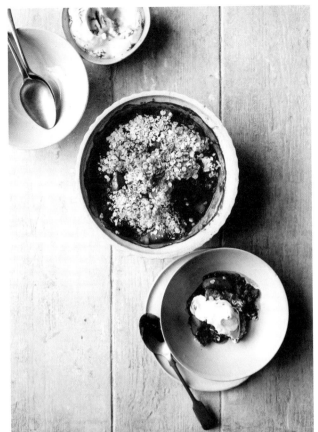

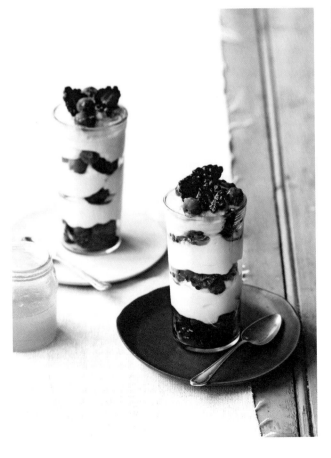

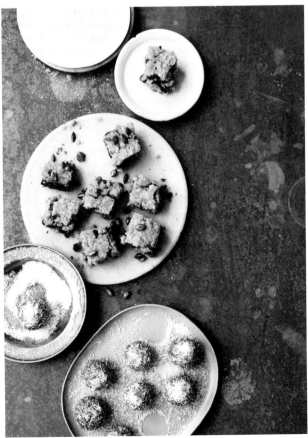

PART 2:

The Recipes

These recipes are designed to introduce you to the possibilities that exist when you decide to commit to healthier eating. Gone are the days of salad and crispbread in the name of eating better. Good, wholesome food can and should be decadent fare. You should be able to enjoy every single meal of the day and not feel that you are signing up for a life of drudgery. I also want to prove to you that eating better does not mean that you have to sell a kidney or remortgage your home, or indeed spend hours in the kitchen knee-deep in pots and pans just to create a nutritious meal.

This is not intended to be an exhaustive resource of healthy recipes. Instead, I want you to get used to the different cooking techniques and what ingredients to use. Eventually you'll be making the most of healthy ingredients instinctively, allowing you to get creative and eat well for life. This is just your introduction to how tasty, easy, accessible and enjoyable healthy eating is. Get your sleeves rolled up, fire up the gas, and get creating!

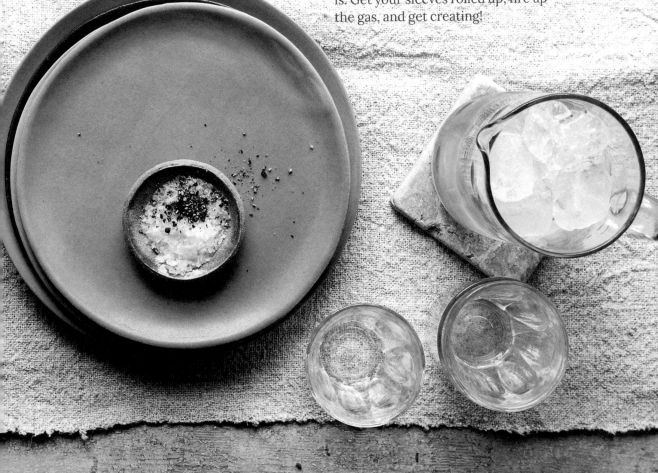

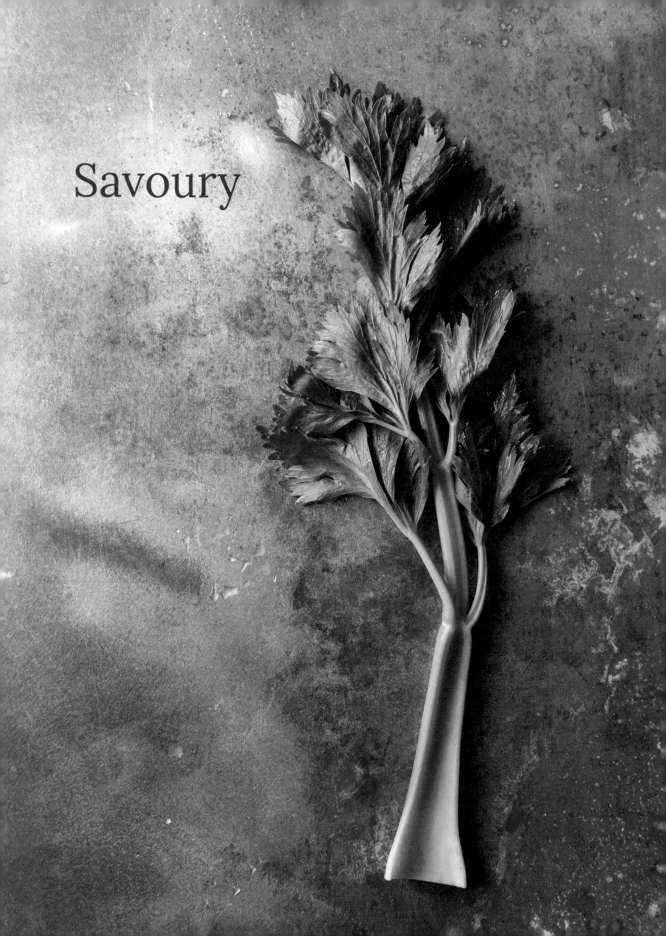

Savoury

Mixed seed houmous

This is a lovely dip that is great with all manner of vegetable crudités, or makes a filling snack when spread on multigrain toast.

Serves: 2–3

300g (10½oz) mixed seeds
4 tablespoons extra virgin olive oil
juice of ½ lemon
1 clove garlic, finely chopped
pinch sea salt

Place the seeds, oil, lemon juice, garlic and salt in a food processor and blitz to a smooth dip. If the mixture seems too thick, add small amounts of water as necessary. Taste and add more salt if needed.

See photograph on page 51.

The best-ever guacamole

I have been making guacamole for years, but I recently went on an incredible trip to Mexico where I tried some amazing variations (including one with crickets in – don't worry, I won't put you through that). Adding a few extras to this simple, good-fat-rich staple takes it up a notch, big time!

Serves: 2–3

2 very ripe avocados
juice of 1 lime
2 tablespoons extra virgin olive oil
1 large clove garlic, finely chopped
1 small red chilli (chile), finely chopped
1 red onion, very finely chopped
150g (5¼oz) pitted green olives,
    roughly chopped
15g (½oz) coriander (cilantro) leaves,
    roughly chopped
sea salt

Scoop all the avocado flesh into a bowl and mash well with a fork. It doesn't have to be completely smooth, as a bit of texture is great here.

Add the lime juice, oil, garlic, chilli (chile), onion, olives and coriander (cilantro), with a generous pinch of salt, and mix well.

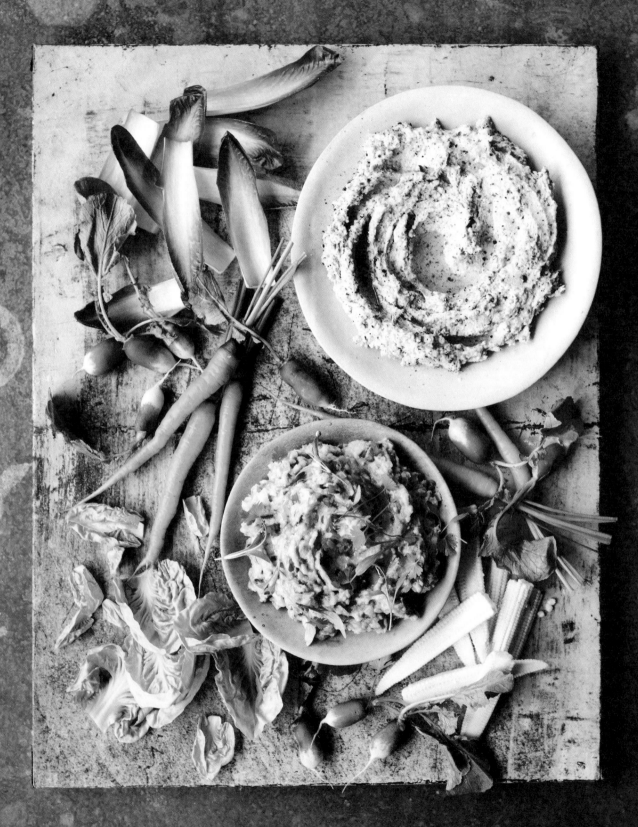

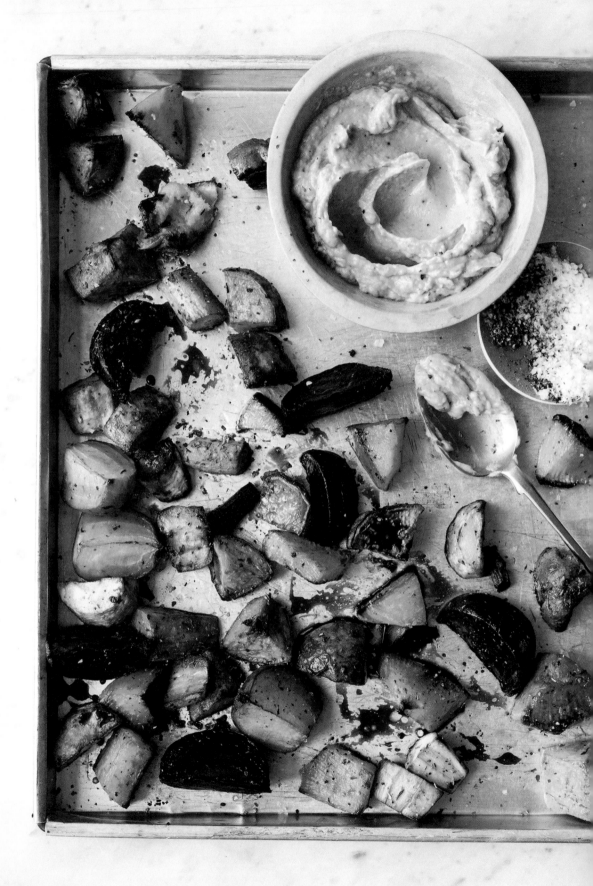

● ROASTING AND BAKING
● GOOD FATS
✗ PERFECT AS A SIDE

Roasted roots with avocado, horseradish and lemon dip

This is a great dish for sharing that can be eaten as a snack or play the lead role in a salad.

Serves: 2–3

2 parsnips
1 large sweet potato
1 beetroot (beet)
½ small swede (rutabaga)
1 tablespoon olive oil
1 tablespoon balsamic vinegar
½ teaspoon garlic granules
½ teaspoon dried mixed herbs
sea salt and black pepper

For the dip
1 large, very ripe avocado
juice of 1 lemon
2 teaspoons hot horseradish sauce

Preheat the oven to 180°C/350°F/Gas mark 4.

Peel all the vegetables, cut them into similar-sized wedges and place in a roasting tray. Drizzle over the oil and balsamic vinegar and sprinkle over the garlic granules, mixed herbs and some salt and pepper. Toss together to mix.

Roast for about 30 minutes until soft, with the edges turning nicely crispy and golden; keep an eye on them as ovens vary.

Meanwhile, scoop the avocado flesh into a blender. Add the lemon juice, horseradish sauce and some salt and pepper, and process to form a smooth dip. Serve with the roasted veg.

Easy homemade dim sum

I absolutely adore dim sum (lunch time in Hong Kong is something I will never forget) and a huge proportion of dim sum are actually steamed. You can make so many amazing varieties by buying ready-made dumpling or wonton skins from a Chinese supermarket or online. Play with all types of fillings and combinations.

Serves: 2

250g (9oz) king prawns (shrimp), ideally
   raw, but cooked are fine, and roughly
   chopped
small bunch coriander (cilantro)
¼ teaspoon minced ginger (storebought,
   or extremely finely chopped)
¼ teaspoon green curry paste
2 spring onions (scallions), finely chopped
16 ready-made wonton/dumpling skins
sea salt

Place the chopped prawns (shrimp) in a bowl and tear the coriander (cilantro) leaves into the bowl. Add the ginger, curry paste, spring onions (scallions) and a pinch of salt, and mix well.

Lay the wonton skins on a dry surface and place a teaspoonful of the prawn mixture in the centre of each. Fold over the skin and pinch the edges together to create a parcel. Prick one side to allow air to circulate and escape.

Place the parcels on an oiled steamer tray and steam for 4–5 minutes, until the prawns are fully cooked.

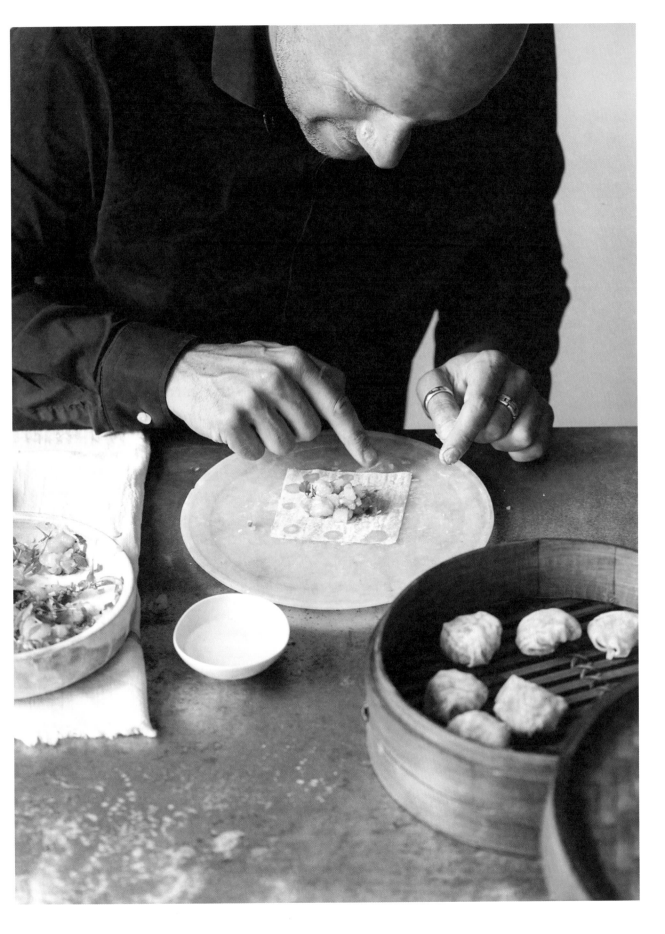

● SWEETS AND SNACKS
● ROASTING AND BAKING
✗ PERFECT AS A SNACK

Kale chips

Kale chips have become a bit of a phenomenon in the last few years but, in all honesty, the prices that many manufacturers charge are beyond a joke – for a bit of dried-up kale! They are super easy and dirt cheap to make yourself.

Serves: 2

500g (1lb 2oz) curly kale
olive oil, for drizzling
sea salt

Preheat the oven to 140°C/275°F/Gas mark 1.

Pick out and discard any of the thicker, woodier stems from the kale.

Drizzle the leaves with olive oil and sprinkle over as much sea salt as you fancy, then toss well to ensure even coverage. Lay the kale in a single layer over several baking sheets (or cook them in batches).

Bake in the oven for around 25 minutes until nice and crispy, keeping an eye on them to make sure they don't burn. Allow to cool completely before storing in an airtight container.

Herbed Parmesan crisps

These are an interesting little snack that can get quite addictive. They are a great low-carb alternative to regular crisps (chips).

Serves: 2

100g (1½ cups) grated Parmesan
    cheese
2 teaspoons dried mixed herbs

Preheat the oven to 200°C/400°F/Gas mark 6 and line a baking sheet with baking parchment.

Mix the Parmesan and dried herbs together well.

Place tablespoons of the cheese mixture on the lined sheet, spacing each heap about 2.5cm (1 inch) or so apart to allow room for them to spread.

Bake for 3–5 minutes until golden. Leave to cool and turn crisp.

See photograph on page 58.

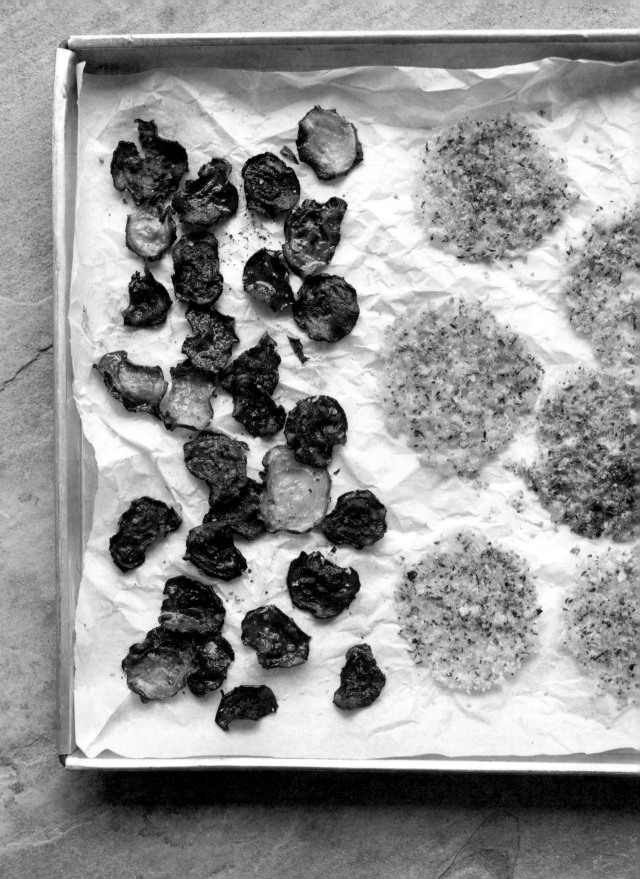

● SWEETS AND SNACKS
● ROASTING AND BAKING
✗ PERFECT AS A SNACK

Balsamic beetroot crisps

I absolutely adore beetroot (beet) crisps. They are super-easy to make and are great on their own or dipped into houmous.

Serves: 2

900g (just over 2lb) beetroot (beet)
2 tablespoons olive oil
1 tablespoon balsamic vinegar
sea salt

Preheat the oven to 150°C/300°F/Gas mark 2.

Wash the beetroot (beets) thoroughly and dry. Cut into very thin slices (think regular crisps [chips]) and place the slices in a bowl.

Mix the oil and balsamic vinegar together and whisk well, then pour over the beetroot slices and toss together well, making sure the slices are completely coated.

Spread the slices out in a single layer on a baking tray (you may need several trays or to do this in batches). Sprinkle a generous pinch of salt over the beetroot and bake for around 30 minutes, or until crisp.

Pear, rocket and Parmesan salad

This is a bit of a classic, and works beautifully with almost anything as a side dish. Fruit and greens can marry together beautifully, and the Parmesan is the culinary glue that brings the pear and rocket (arugula) together so well.

Serves: 1

1 ripe pear
45g (1½oz) rocket (arugula)
3–4 teaspoons shaved Parmesan
  cheese

For the dressing
1 teaspoon apple cider vinegar
1 tablespoon olive oil
sea salt and black pepper

Cut the pear lengthways into 8 slices, discarding any pips.

Place the rocket (arugula) on a plate. Fan the pear slices out on top of it and sprinkle the Parmesan over the top.

Whisk together the dressing ingredients, with salt and pepper to taste, and dress the salad to serve.

Brown rice salad

This is a great side dish, and it is also a good way to use up leftover vegetables and bits and pieces in the fridge. Any combination works really well, but it is especially good with fish, chicken or even with a vegetable curry.

Serves: 2

150g (¾ cup) brown rice
1 teaspoon vegetable bouillon powder
1 spring onion (scallion), thinly sliced
  lengthways
1 carrot, cut into thin matchsticks
handful spinach leaves, shredded
sea salt and black pepper

Place the rice and bouillon powder in a saucepan. Cover with boiling water and simmer for around 20 minutes, or until the rice is soft. Drain.

Toss the prepared vegetables through the drained rice and finish with some salt and pepper.

Butternut, beetroot and red onion balsamic with salsa verde

This is an amazing side dish that packs in some pretty bold flavours and boasts crazy colours when you serve it up. Its sharp and earthy tastes make it great with anything from game meat to vegetarian bakes, or even as part of a warm salad. Try adding some goat cheese for extra zing if you want it!

Serves: 2

½ small butternut squash, diced and seeded, skin left on
2 large, raw beetroot (beets), scrubbed then diced, skins left on (to retain that important fibre)
1 large red onion, peeled and cut into wedges
olive oil, for drizzling
2 tablespoons balsamic vinegar
sea salt and black pepper

For the salsa verde:

½ clove garlic, finely chopped
2 handfuls flat-leaf parsley
handful basil
handful mint
2 teaspoons capers
2 anchovies
2 teaspoons apple cider vinegar
2 tablespoons olive oil

Preheat the oven to 180°C/350°F/Gas mark 4.

Put the diced vegetables and onion on a baking sheet. Drizzle with olive oil, 1 tablespoon of the balsamic vinegar, plus a pinch of salt and pepper. Roast for about 30 minutes, or until soft with the edges browning. Turn the vegetables occasionally, and halfway through the cooking time, add the second tablespoon of balsamic vinegar.

To make the salsa verde, add all ingredients to a food processor and pulse to a coarse salsa.

Serve the roasted vegetables with a drizzle of the salsa over the top.

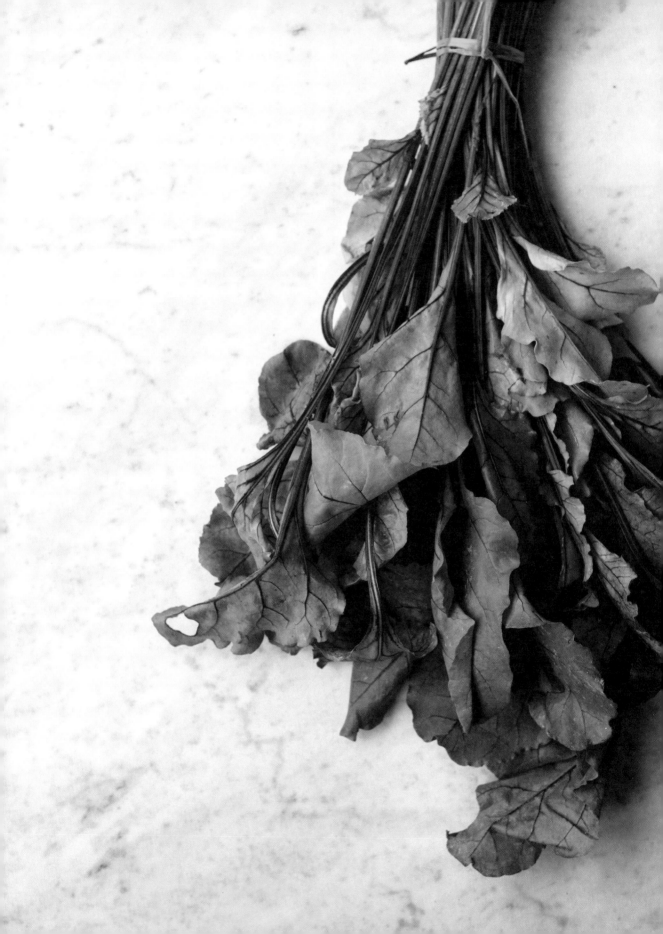

Killer kale salad

I know, I know, the prospect of eating raw kale is about as exciting as watching paint dry. But, with a little bit of creativity, raw kale can be an amazing base for a salad. I swear to you, I have used variations of these flavours and had vegetable dodgers the land over coming back for seconds!

Serves: 2

1 small sweet potato, diced
   (skin left on)
olive oil, for drizzling
200g (7oz) curly kale
1 red (bell) pepper, diced
5 cherry tomatoes, quartered
sea salt

For the dressing
1 large clove garlic, finely chopped
1 small red chilli (chile), finely chopped
1 teaspoon honey
2 teaspoons light soy sauce
1 heaped tablespoon almond butter
½ teaspoon Chinese five-spice powder
small handful coriander (cilantro)
   leaves, roughly chopped

Preheat the oven to 200°C/400°F/Gas mark 6.

Place the sweet potato in a roasting tray, drizzle with a little olive oil and a small sprinkling of salt, and roast for about 20 minutes, turning occasionally, until soft and the edges are turning golden. Remove and set aside.

Place the kale in a bowl, drizzle with a little olive oil, then get your hands in there and give it a good massage. Keep this up until it softens, wilts, and starts to resemble cooked kale.

Add the (bell) pepper, tomatoes and roasted sweet potato, and toss well.

For the dressing, put the garlic and chilli (chile) in a small bowl, then add the honey and soy, followed by the almond butter and five-spice. Mix well. Add 1 tablespoon water and mix well again. Add another 1 tablespoon water and the chopped coriander (cilantro) and mix well. The dressing should be a smooth, creamy texture, not too thick or too watery. Dress the vegetables to serve.

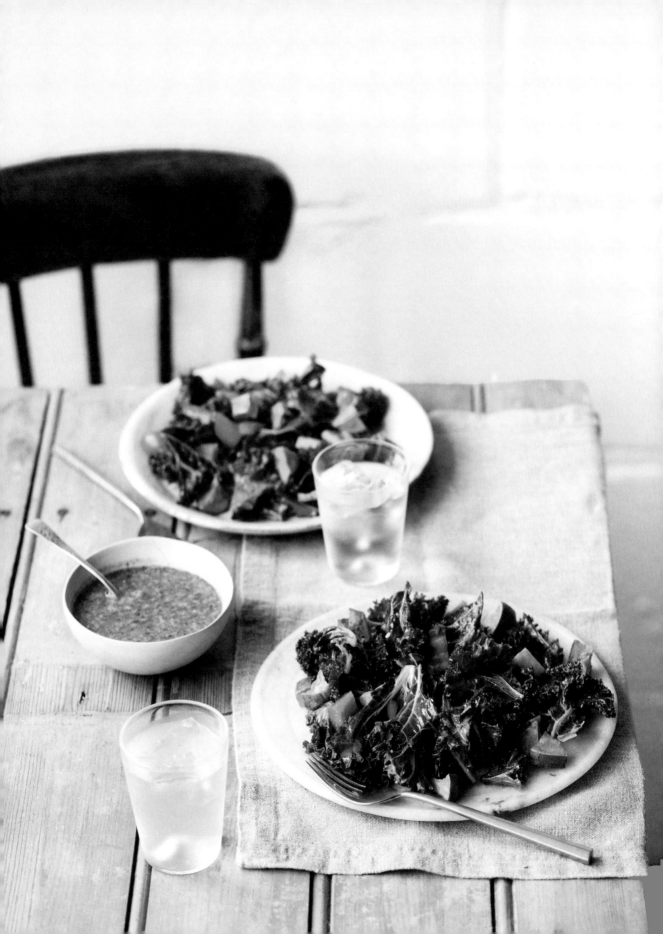

Carrot "noodle" salad

There certainly seems to be a real craze of late for vegetable noodles and things of that ilk. These aren't anything new, though: I remember chowing down on spiralized sweet potato noodles back in the 1990s. Making vegetable noodles is a great way of bringing new textures into salads; we have all had chopped and sliced vegetables a million times, but getting creative with shape and texture makes things interesting again. In this recipe I have opted for a vegetable peeler to make flat noodles. If you have a spiralizer, then by all means use it for this.

Serves: 1 for lunch or 2 as a side

2 large carrots
1 teaspoon olive oil
2 spring onions (scallions)
1 teaspoon raisins
2 teaspoons sesame seeds
small bunch coriander
  (cilantro), torn

For the dressing
1 teaspoon honey
1 clove garlic, finely chopped or crushed
½ teaspoon curry powder
1 teaspoon light soy sauce
4 teaspoons extra virgin olive oil

Using a swivel vegetable peeler, slice down the length of the carrots to give long, thin ribbons that resemble flat noodles. Place these in a bowl and drizzle over the olive oil. Toss well, then set aside for 10 minutes.

Cut the spring onions (scallions) on the diagonal into long slices then add to the carrots with the raisins, sesame seeds and torn coriander (cilantro).

Combine all the dressing ingredients and whisk well. Dress the salad and toss.

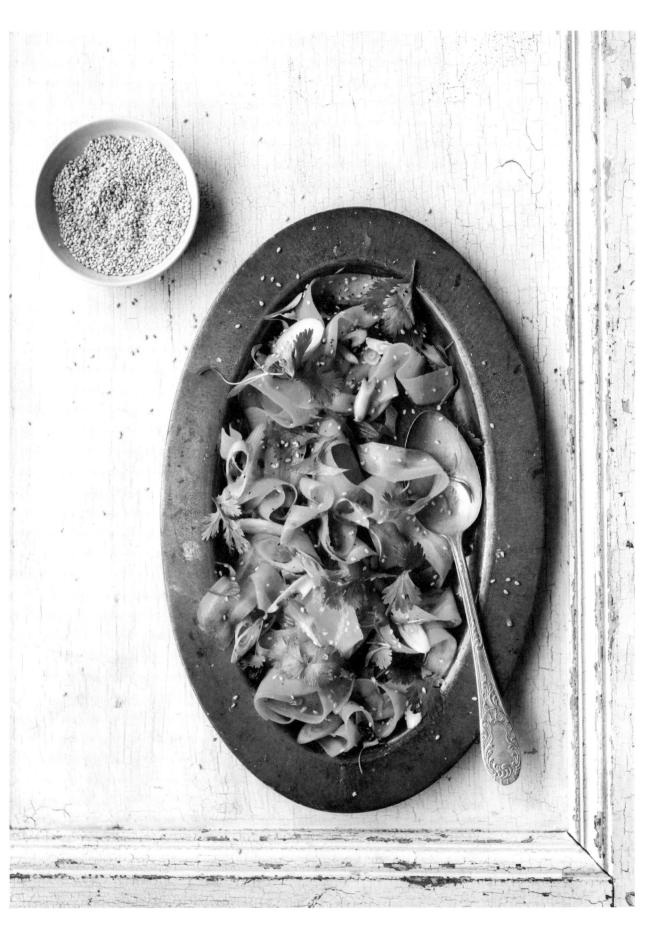

● SALADS
● GOOD FATS
● FISH AND SEAFOOD
✗ PERFECT AS A LIGHT LUNCH

Avocado and smoked salmon salad

This is a lovely, super-simple way of getting your good fats in. Crisp and satisfying.

Serves: 2

1 large, ripe avocado, halved
juice of ½ lemon
2 teaspoons wasabi paste (less if you
   don't like it too hot)
3 handfuls mixed salad leaves
5 cherry tomatoes, halved
80g (2¾oz) smoked salmon,
   thinly sliced
sea salt and black pepper

Scoop the flesh of one half of the avocado into a small food processor along with the lemon juice, wasabi, 2 tablespoons water (or a little more to make it runnier) and salt and pepper to taste. Blitz to a smooth, creamy, pourable dressing.

Dice the remaining avocado half. Combine the salad leaves, tomatoes, smoked salmon and diced avocado on a plate and dress with the avocado wasabi dressing.

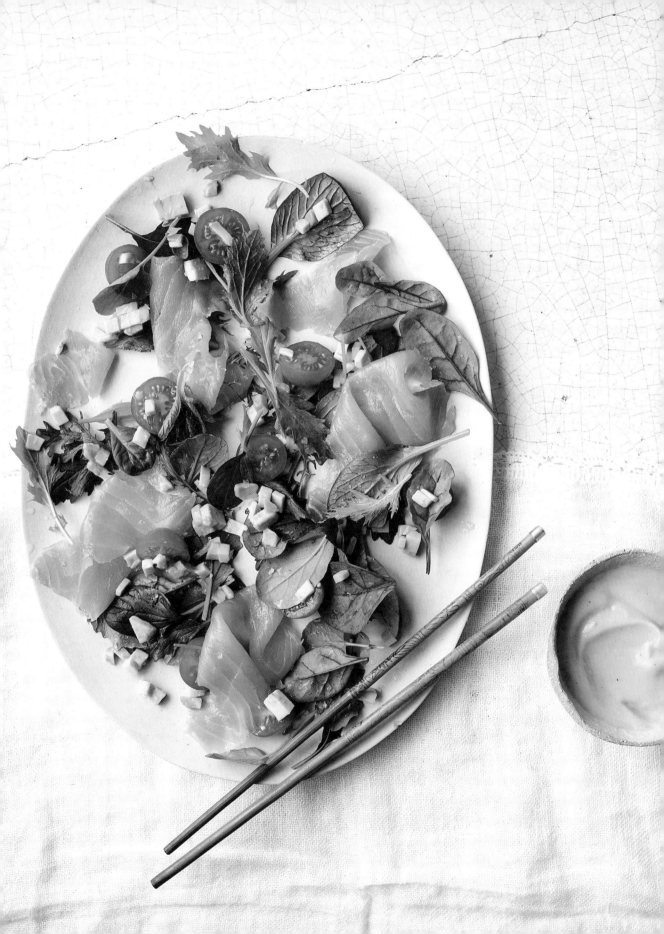

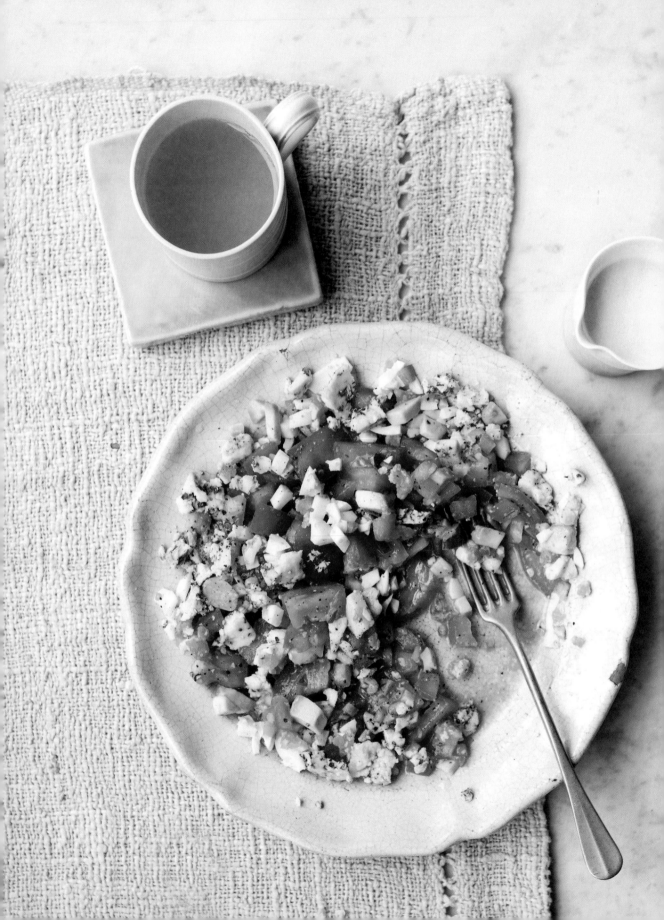

● SALADS
● GOOD FATS
✗ PERFECT FOR LUNCH

Cheeky chopped salad

Packed with protein, good fats, minerals and phytochemicals, this is the perfect salad for protein junkies. It will keep you full for hours.

Serves: 1

1 ripe avocado, finely diced
2 large tomatoes, finely diced
¼ red onion, finely diced
2 hard-boiled eggs, finely diced
50g (1¾oz) blue cheese, finely diced
   or crumbled
sea salt and black pepper

For the Parmesan cream
80g (1¼ cups) freshly grated Parmesan
   cheese
½ clove garlic, finely chopped
   or crushed
1 teaspoon horseradish sauce

Combine the avocado, tomatoes and red onion in a bowl, and toss with a pinch each of salt and pepper. Transfer to a serving plate and top with the diced egg and blue cheese.

Whisk together the Parmesan cream ingredients with 2–3 tablespoons water and dress the salad with the cream.

Honey mustard, watercress and radish salad

This is a great salad for fiery flavours, with a wonderful spectrum of nutrients added to boot. The cucumber and fennel offer contrast to the pepperiness, adding a cooling quality. With the sweetness of the dressing, this salad gives three interesting flavour hits in one.

Serves: 2

50g (1¾oz) watercress
2 handfuls baby spinach leaves
4–5 radishes, sliced
½ cucumber, cut into batons
½ fennel bulb, cut into thin matchsticks

For the dressing
2 teaspoons honey
1 teaspoon English mustard
1 teaspoon light soy sauce
1 tablespoon olive oil

Combine all the salad ingredients together in a bowl.

Mix the dressing ingredients well to form a smooth, golden dressing. Dress the salad and toss well.

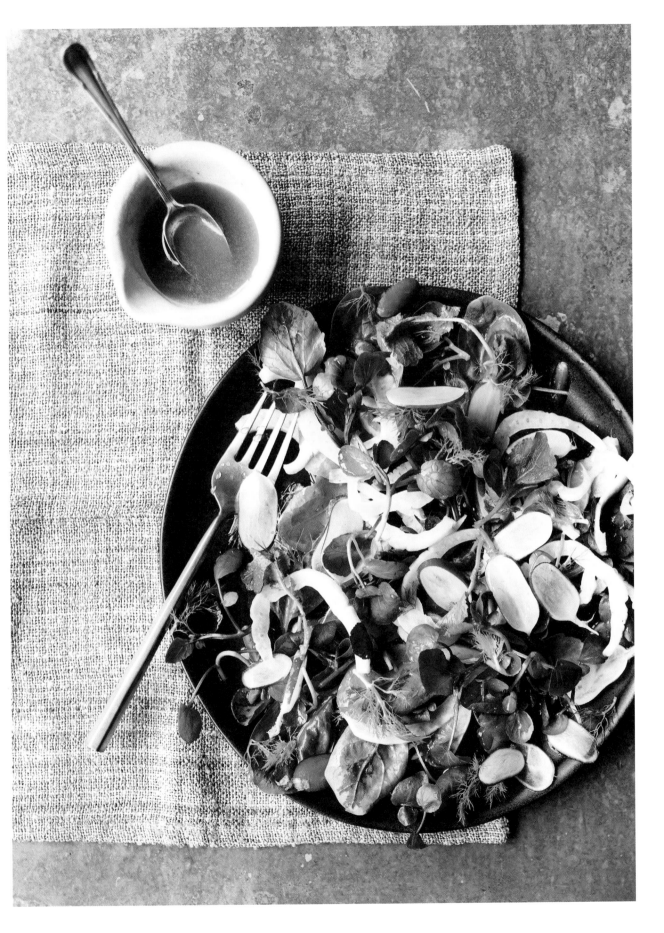

Grilled corn, avocado, coriander and red chilli salad

This is a beautiful salad with a real Mexican flair. So many flavours and textures, and with them comes a wonderful array of important nutrients.

Serves: 1 for lunch or 2 as a side

1 large corn on the cob, leaves stripped
3 handfuls mixed salad leaves
1 large, ripe avocado, diced
1 x 400g (14oz) can black beans, drained
small bunch coriander (cilantro)
1 large red chilli (chile), sliced

For the dressing
juice of 1 lime
1 teaspoon honey
1 tablespoon extra virgin olive oil

Heat a griddle pan over a high heat until very hot. Place the corn cob in the pan and allow to cook for 3–4 minutes before turning. Repeat to ensure a gentle charring all over. Remove the charred cob from the pan and leave until cool enough to handle. Stand the cob upright on a board and use a knife to slice down the length of the cob, close to the core, to liberate the individual kernels.

Place the salad leaves in a bowl. Add the charred corn kernels, avocado, black beans, coriander (cilantro) and chilli (chile), and toss together well.

Mix all the dressing ingredients together and dress the salad, before tossing well again.

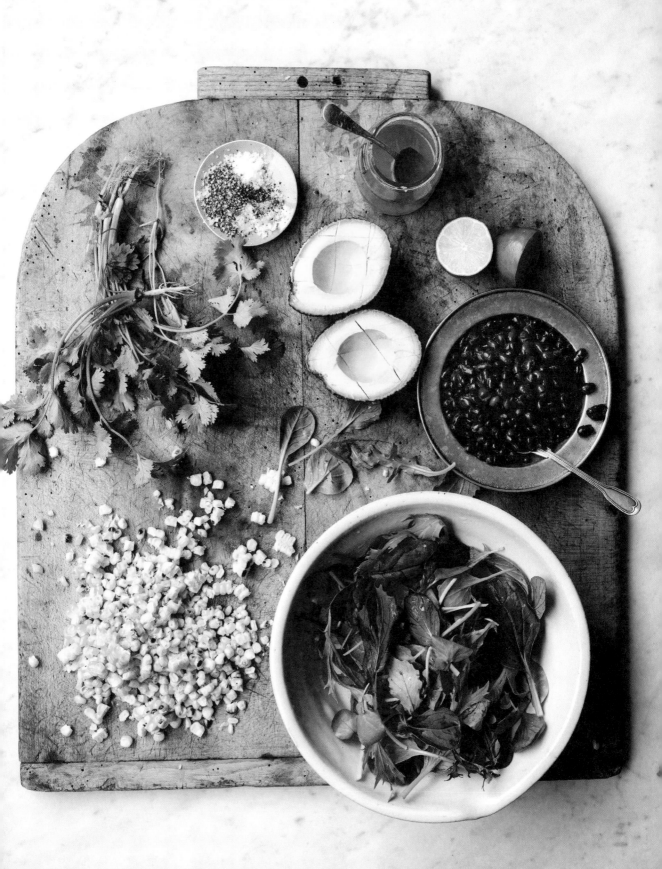

Roasted fennel, green pea and rocket salad with goat cheese

This is a beautiful, vibrant, summery salad. Roasting vegetables and throwing them into salads can be so successful; the contrast of warm and cool is great. Fennel roasts beautifully.

Serves: 1 for lunch or 2 as a side

1 fennel bulb
olive oil, for drizzling
45g (1½oz) rocket (arugula)
2 handfuls frozen garden peas,
 defrosted
60g (2oz) soft goat cheese
sea salt and black pepper

Preheat the oven to 200°C/400°F/Gas mark 6.

Slice the fennel bulb into quarters lengthways, leaving the root intact so that the layers of each quarter hold together, and put into a roasting tray or dish. Drizzle with a little olive oil, sprinkle over a pinch each of salt and pepper and roast for 20–25 minutes until soft and turning golden brown at the edges; keep checking to avoid burning.

Combine the rocket (arugula), peas and roasted fennel in a bowl. Crumble over the goat cheese and sprinkle over some cracked black pepper and a pinch of salt. Toss well.

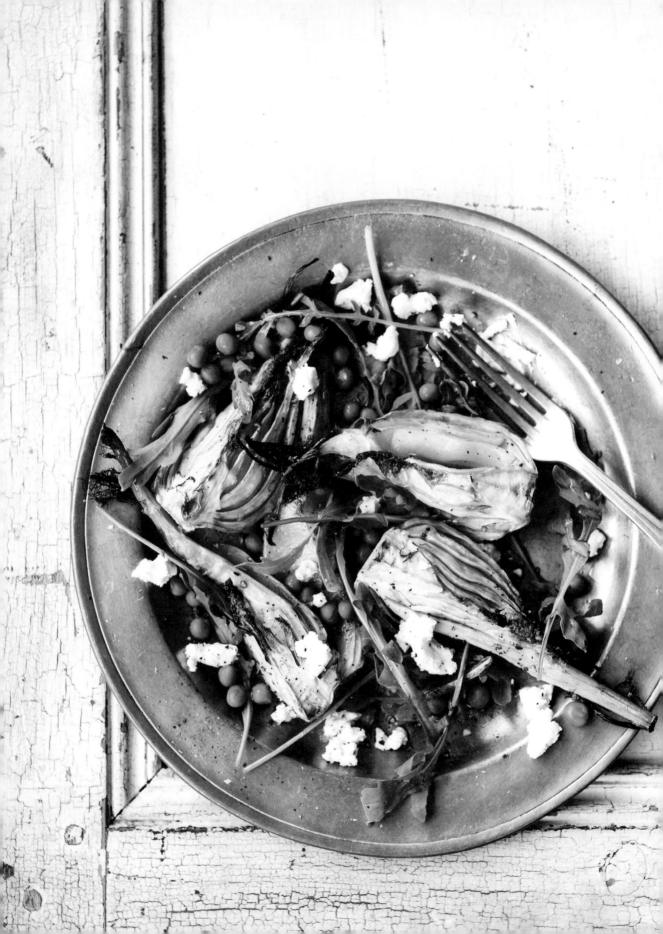

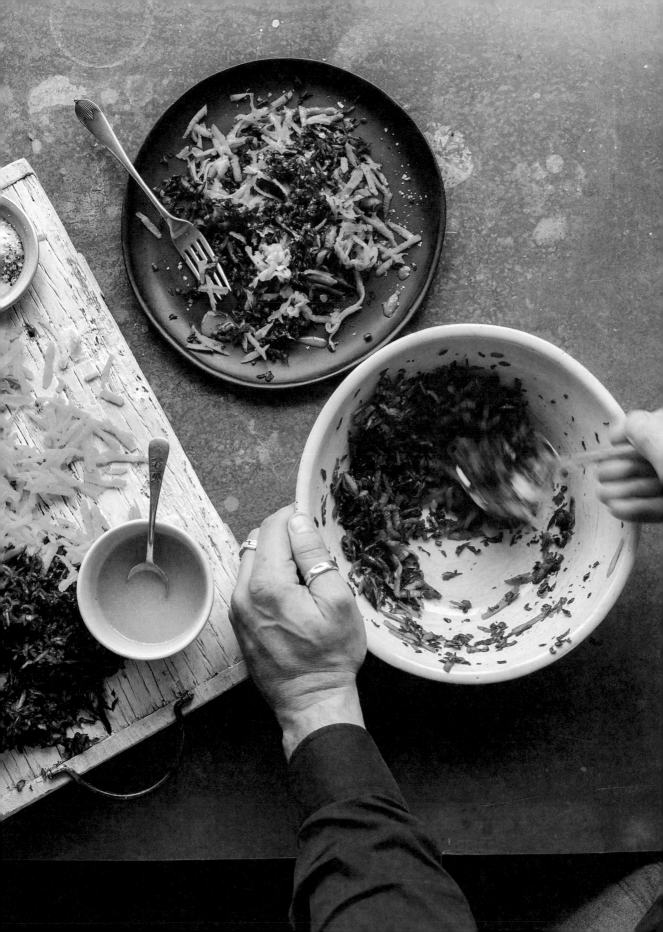

Carrot, apple and red cabbage sesame salad

This is a serious flavour bomb and is as much at home in a bun with a burger as it is served as an accompaniment. It's great with cheeses or oily fish, and amazing with vegetarian curries and stews.

Serves: 2–3

¼ large red cabbage
1 large, sharp apple
   (Granny Smith is ideal)
2 large carrots
1 tablespoon sesame seeds

For the dressing
1 heaped teaspoon miso paste
1 teaspoon honey
½ teaspoon mustard
2 teaspoons toasted sesame oil

Grate the cabbage, apple and carrots into a bowl.

Place all the dressing ingredients with 2 teaspoons water in small bowl and mix together thoroughly. The dressing should have a smooth, creamy consistency, so add a little more water only if necessary.

Dress the grated vegetables and toss well. Sprinkle the sesame seeds over the salad before serving.

Savoury vegetable quinoa

This is a great accompaniment to such a wide variety of dishes. It is ideal in the summer served cold at a barbecue, alongside cold meats and salads, or to take on a picnic. It is also really good served hot with stews, roasted meats and vegetarian dishes.

Serves: 2

100g (heaped ½ cup) quinoa
1 teaspoon vegetable bouillon powder
olive oil, for cooking
½ red onion, finely chopped
1 clove garlic, finely chopped
1 small courgette (zucchini), finely diced
1 red (bell) pepper, finely diced
2 handfuls curly kale, torn or chopped
   into very small pieces
sea salt and black pepper

Place the quinoa and bouillon powder in a saucepan and cover with boiling water. Simmer for around 20 minutes until cooked (it will soften and a small tail-like projection will appear on the side). Drain and set aside.

Heat a little oil in a large frying pan, add the onion, garlic, courgette (zucchini), (bell) pepper and a generous pinch of salt and sauté until all the vegetables have softened.

Add the kale and sauté for another minute, before adding the drained quinoa. Mix thoroughly and season to taste with salt and pepper.

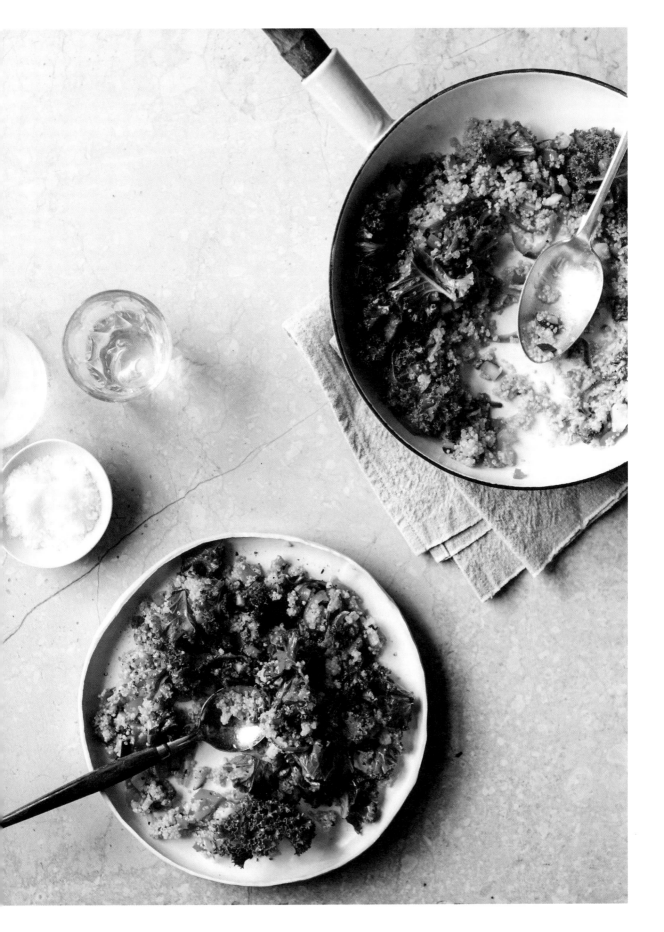

Courgette-topped baked pilaf

This is a bit of a special dish. It is based on something I once ate at a vegetarian restaurant in Cyprus, to which I've added my own slant. The combination of courgette (zucchini) and cinnamon is really quite magical in this type of cuisine.

Serves: 2

olive oil, for cooking
3–4 large courgettes (zucchini),
    cut lengthways into 5mm
    (¼ inch) slices
1 red onion, peeled, halved
    and thinly sliced
1 clove garlic, finely chopped

150g (¾ cup) short-grain brown rice
½ teaspoon ground cinnamon
8 dried apricots, diced
3 tablespoons cashew nuts
about 500ml (generous 2 cups)
    vegetable stock
3 handfuls baby spinach
sea salt and black pepper

Preheat the oven to 150°C/300°F/Gas mark 2.

Heat a little oil in a large frying pan and fry the long courgette (zucchini) slices until soft and completely malleable. Season well and set aside.

Heat a little oil in a separate pan, add the onion and garlic and sauté until soft. Add the rice, cinnamon, apricots, cashews and half the vegetable stock, and allow to simmer until the rice is cooked. Keep topping up with stock if it begins to dry out before the rice is cooked. Just before the rice is cooked, add the spinach and allow to wilt. You want it to cook to the point where the rice is soft and fully cooked, but there is no noticeable liquid left in the pan.

Use the cooked courgette slices to line the base and sides of a small, round baking or casserole dish, so that the slices overhang the edge of the dish. Spoon the rice mixture into the courgette-lined dish, press down to pack it in, and fold any overhanging courgette slices back over the top to cover.

Bake for about 25 minutes, then remove from the oven. Place a tray over the top of the dish, and flip it over. Gently pull the dish off and slice like a cake to serve.

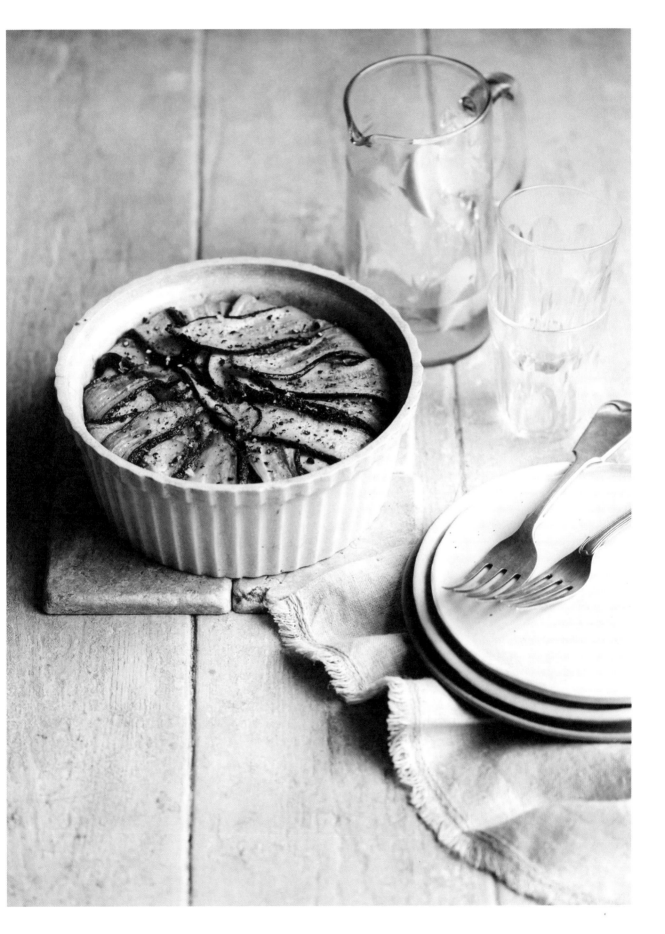

Aubergine stuffed with tomato and spinach quinoa

This is a lovely, flavoursome dish that is very filling and satisfying.
Great with salad or sautéed greens.

Serves: 2

100g (heaped ½ cup) quinoa
1 large aubergine (eggplant)
olive oil, for cooking
1 large red onion, finely chopped

2 cloves garlic, finely chopped
500g (1lb 2oz) passata (strained
  tomatoes)
2 handfuls baby spinach
100g (3½oz) feta cheese
sea salt

Preheat the oven to 180°C/350°F/Gas mark 4.

Place the quinoa in a saucepan and cover with boiling water. Simmer for around 20 minutes, or until it is cooked (it will soften and a small tail-like projection will appear on the side). Drain and set aside.

Cut the aubergine (eggplant) in half lengthways and scoop out the flesh from the skin, taking care to leave the skin intact. Cut the flesh into dice and set aside. Place the scooped-out skins on a baking tray, hollow side down, and add a little water to the tray. Bake at the top of the oven for about 15 minutes, then turn them over and bake for another 10 minutes.

Meanwhile, heat a little oil in a pan, add the onion, garlic and a pinch of salt and sauté until the onion has softened. Add the diced aubergine flesh and the passata (strained tomatoes) and simmer for 15 minutes, stirring frequently, until the aubergine is cooked and the passata has reduced to a thick sauce.

Add the drained quinoa to the tomato and aubergine mixture, and mix well. Simmer for 4–5 minutes, then throw in the spinach and continue to cook until the spinach wilts. Spoon the quinoa mixture into the aubergine skins, crumble over the feta and bake for another 10 minutes.

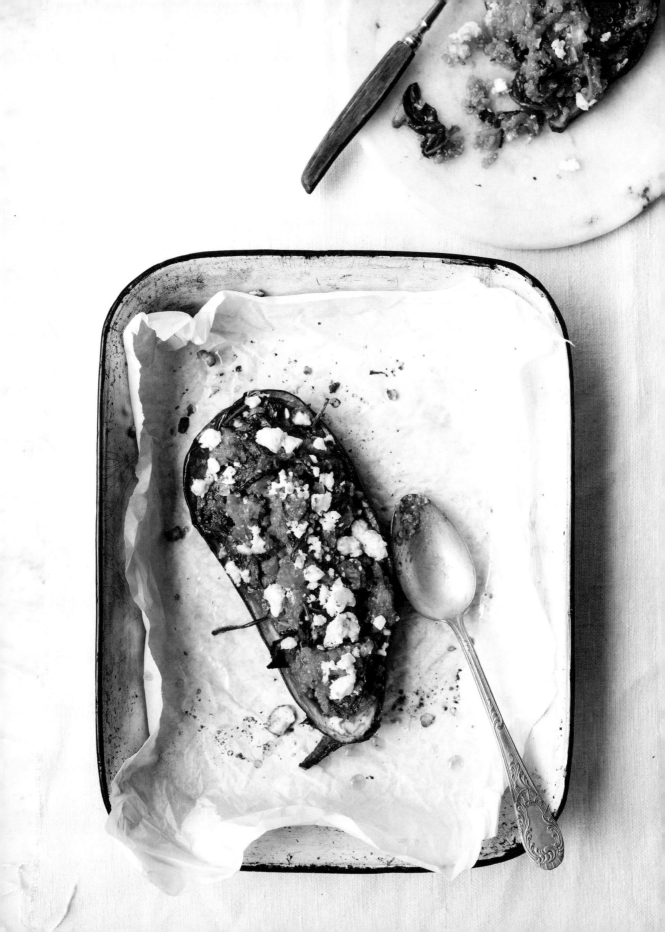

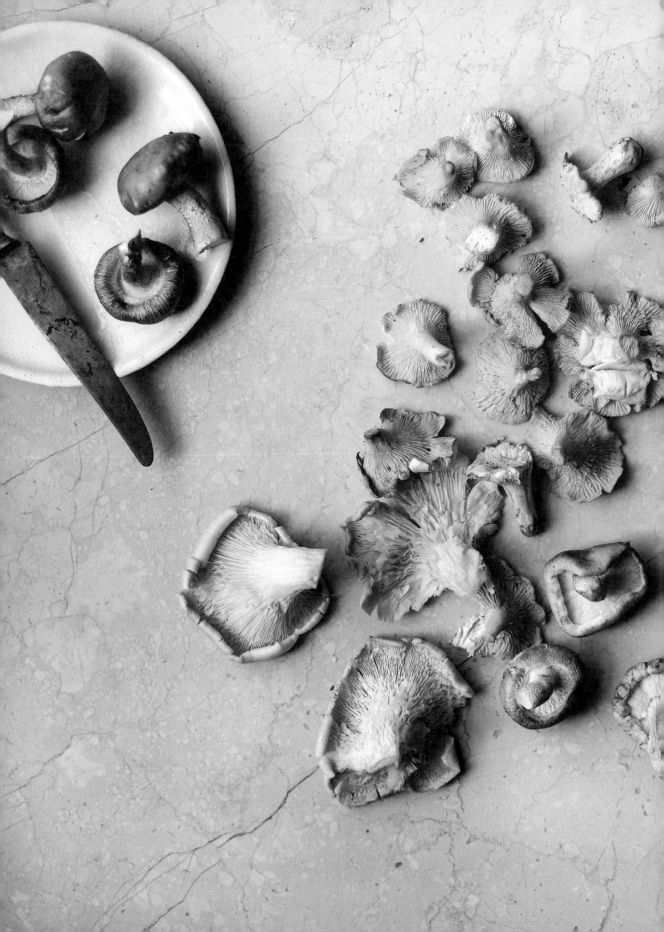

Wild mushroom and rosemary barley risotto

I do love a good risotto. The problem is, regular risotto rice is very refined and is a bit of a blood sugar bomb, so I would advise anyone trying to build a healthier diet to give it a wide berth. Swapping arborio rice for pearl barley creates an amazing risotto that has a great texture, a nutty flavour and, best of all, offers all the health benefits associated with dense whole grains.

Serves: 2

olive oil, for cooking
1 large white onion, finely sliced
2 cloves garlic, finely sliced
2 large sprigs rosemary
250g (1⅓ cups) pearl barley
20g (¾oz) dried porcini mushrooms

500ml (generous 2 cups) chicken stock
200g (7oz) fresh mixed wild mushrooms (any combination you can find), roughly chopped
2 tablespoons cream cheese
sea salt and black pepper

Heat a little oil in a pan, add the onion, garlic, rosemary and a pinch of salt and sauté until the onion has softened.

Add the pearl barley and the dried porcini mushrooms, with just a small amount of the stock.

Simmer, stirring, and keep adding the stock a little at a time, as needed, until the barley has softened and the mixture begins to turn a little creamy, like a regular risotto. If you need more liquid, a little hot water will do.

Add the chopped wild mushrooms and continue to simmer for around 5 minutes, until the mushrooms are cooked.

Remove the rosemary sprigs, stir in the cream cheese and season to taste with salt and pepper before serving.

Classic tabbouleh

Tabbouleh is one of my absolute favourite side dishes. It is so zingy and vibrant, and has a serious amount of nutrients in it from the herbs. Perfect as part of a salad, or as a side to Mediterranean dishes, especially grilled halloumi or falafel.

Serves: 1 for lunch or 2 as a side

25g (1oz) bulgur wheat
1 large tomato, diced
large bunch flat-leaf parsley,
   roughly chopped
small bunch mint, roughly chopped
1 small red onion, finely chopped
2 teaspoons capers
juice of ½ lemon
juice of ½ lime
3 tablespoons olive oil
sea salt and black pepper

Place the bulgur wheat in a saucepan and cover with boiling water. Simmer for around 25 minutes, until the wheat has enlarged and softened. Drain and allow to cool for a few minutes, then transfer to a bowl.

Add the remaining ingredients with salt and pepper to taste, and toss together well.

Barley and roasted squash salad with blue cheese and walnuts

This is an amazing grain-based salad, with multiple textures. It can be a main course in its own right, as well as a side.

Serves: 2

150g (scant ¾ cup) pearl barley
½ small butternut squash,
   seeded and diced (skin left on)
olive oil, for cooking
5 cherry tomatoes, halved
¼ ripe avocado, diced
1 spring onion (scallion), finely sliced

large handful rocket (arugula)
2 tablespoons walnut halves
80g (2¾oz) blue cheese

For the dressing
1 tablespoon orange juice
1 tablespoon olive oil
sea salt and black pepper

Preheat the oven to 180°C/350°F/Gas mark 4.

Place the pearl barley in a saucepan and cover with boiling water. Simmer for 20–25 minutes until cooked and fluffy. Drain well and transfer to a salad bowl.

Meanwhile, place the diced squash in a roasting tray, drizzle a little oil over and roast in the oven for about 20 minutes until soft, with the edges turning golden brown.

Add the tomatoes, avocado, spring onion (scallion), rocket (arugula), walnuts and roasted squash to the drained barley, and toss well.

Mix the orange juice and oil for the dressing together, with salt and pepper to taste, and dress the salad, then toss well again. Crumble the blue cheese over the top to serve.

Minted quinoa and feta burgers

These make a great little alternative to meat burgers: crunchy, rich and filling. I love them with a salad and they work really well in buns too, like a regular burger.

Makes: 4–6

250g (1½ cups) quinoa
2 eggs, beaten
2 teaspoons dried oregano
small bunch mint, finely chopped
1 clove garlic, finely chopped
120g (4¼oz) feta cheese, crumbled
olive oil, for frying
black pepper

Place the quinoa in a saucepan and cover with boiling water. Simmer for around 20 minutes, or until it is cooked (it will soften and a small tail-like projection will appear on the side). Pour into a sieve and set aside to drain.

In a bowl, mix the drained quinoa with the eggs, oregano, mint, garlic, feta and pepper to taste. The mixture should stick together when squeezed. Shape into 4-6 patties.

Fry the patties in a little olive oil for 4 minutes each side, or until golden and crispy.

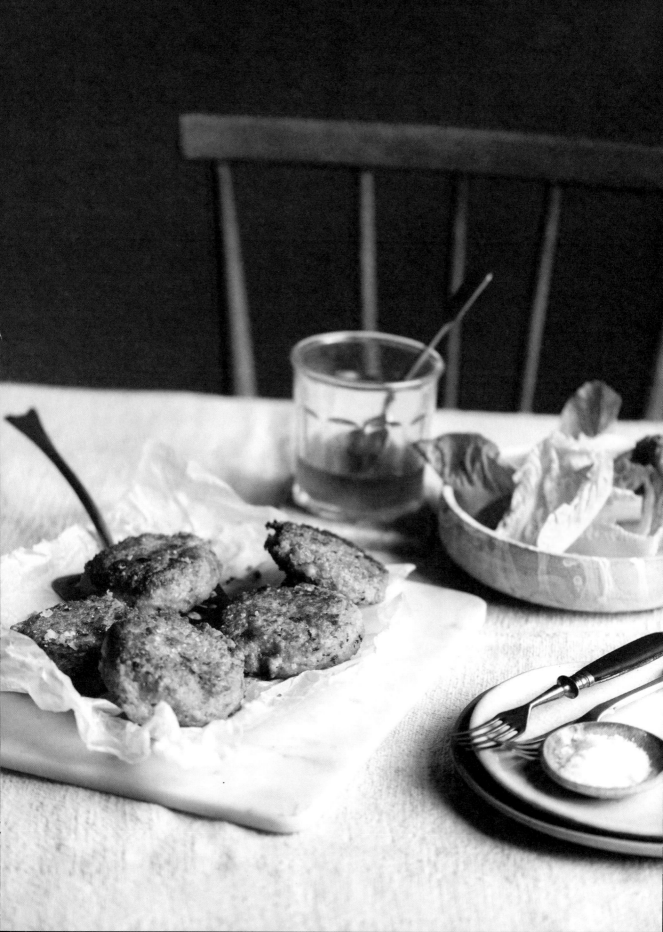

Asian-style coconut rice

I absolutely adore coconut rice, and this makes a fantastic accompaniment to a whole range of Asian dishes, such as Sticky Chilli Chicken and Greens on page 128. It's also amazing with Thai curries, seafood dishes and Indian dhals.

Serves: 2

150g (¾ cup) brown basmati rice
400ml (1¾ cups) coconut milk
1 tablespoon desiccated (dried
   shredded) coconut
1 teaspoon light soy sauce

Place all the ingredients in a saucepan and bring to a simmer. The coconut milk will rapidly reduce as it is absorbed by the rice, so keep topping up with small amounts of water (3–4 tablespoons maximum) then continue simmering until it reduces again, then repeat. Keep this going for about 20 minutes, or until the rice is soft.

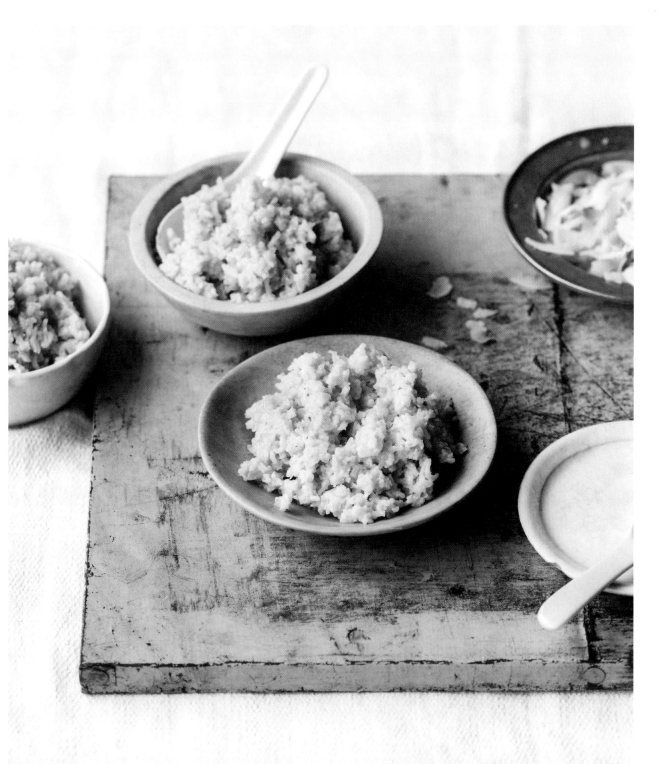

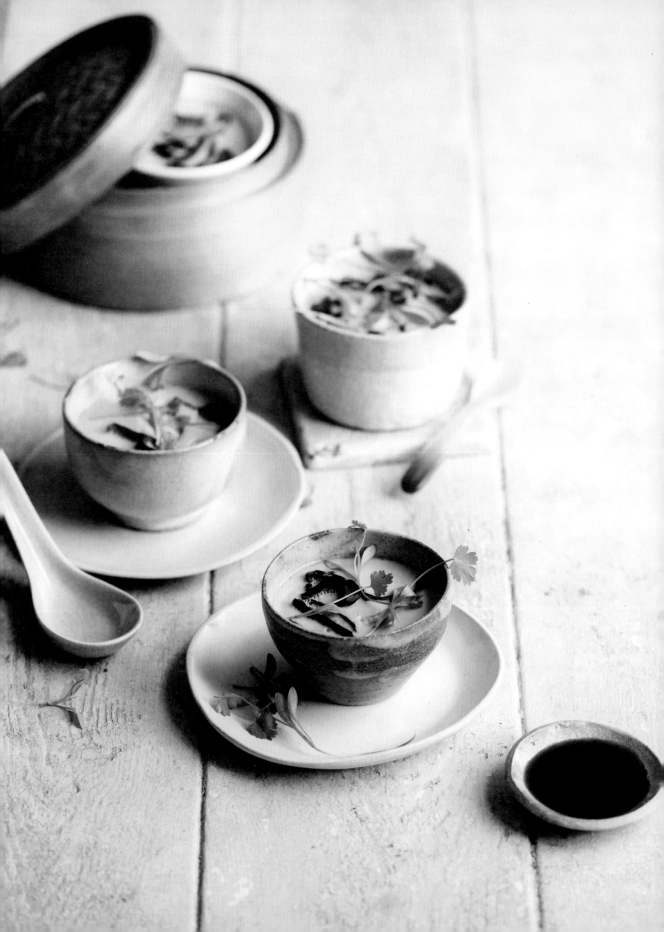

Chawanmushi

This awesome savoury egg custard is a Japanese speciality, and on my first visit to Japan when I tried it, I wasn't quite sure what it was. However, it has a lovely flavour and texture. You could throw all manner of vegetables and seafood into this dish. Dashi stock is available in Asian supermarkets, but if you can't find it, use vegetable stock instead.

Serves: 4

4 shiitake mushrooms, sliced in half
olive oil, for frying
3 eggs
240ml (1 cup) dashi stock
1 teaspoon dark soy sauce
1 teaspoon cooking sake (optional)
4 large, cooked king prawns (shrimp)
coriander (cilantro), to serve
sea salt

Briefly sauté the shiitake mushrooms in olive oil and allow to cool completely.

Crack the eggs into a bowl and beat well.

In a separate bowl, combine the stock, soy sauce, sake, if using, and a pinch of salt. Mix well then begin to add this mixture to the eggs, beating as you go to ensure an even mix.

Place two slices of mushroom and one prawn (shrimp) in each of 4 cups. Fill the cups with the egg mixture.

Place the cups in a steamer and steam for around 15 minutes. Check that they are cooked by inserting a toothpick into them; if it comes out with egg mixture on it, then steam for a bit longer. Garnish with coriander (cilantro) to serve.

Tofu, broccoli and almond Thai-style stir-fry

This is a gorgeous lunch dish that can work perfectly on its own as a light lunch, or with rice or quinoa for something more substantial.

Serves: 2

olive oil, for cooking
2 lemongrass stalks, bashed
  with a rolling pin
2 star anise
2 cloves garlic, finely chopped
100g (3½oz) Tenderstem
  (long-stemmed) broccoli
2 spring onions (scallions), sliced
  on the diagonal into long shreds
80g (2¾oz) marinated or plain firm
  tofu (bean curd), cubed
2 teaspoons honey
2 teaspoons fish sauce
juice of ¼ lime
1 tablespoon whole almonds

Heat a little oil in a wok or large saucepan. Add the bashed lemongrass stalks and star anise and stir-fry for 2–3 minutes until the scent of the lemongrass is released. Add the garlic and broccoli and stir-fry for around 5 minutes, until the broccoli is a brighter green and is starting to soften.

Add the spring onions (scallions) and tofu (bean curd) and continue to stir-fry for another 3 minutes. Add the honey, fish sauce and lime juice and simmer until the sauce caramelizes a little. Add the almonds and serve.

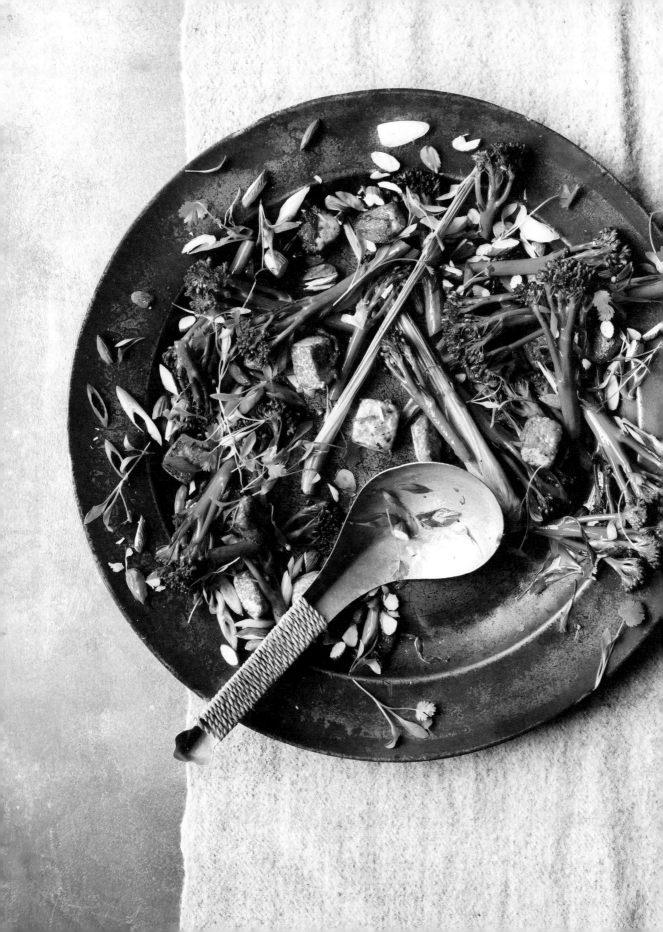

Spinach-stuffed tomatoes

These are so versatile! They make a great breakfast, lunch, little side dish or the focal point of a salad. Great for al fresco summer dining and barbecues: fresh, vibrant and tasty.

Serves: 2–3

300g (10½oz) cooked spinach
  (defrosted frozen or lightly
  steamed fresh)
1 large egg
1 tablespoon full-fat cream cheese
pinch nutmeg
6 large tomatoes (beef [beef steak]
  tomatoes work well)
sea salt and black pepper

Ensure that as much moisture as possible is squeezed from the spinach, especially if you have just steamed it yourself. Once as dry as possible, place in a bowl.

Whisk the egg and cream cheese together then add to the spinach and mix thoroughly. Stir in the nutmeg and some salt and pepper.

Cut the tops off the tomatoes and scoop out and discard the insides. Fill the tomatoes with the spinach mixture, place in a steamer and steam for around 20 minutes.

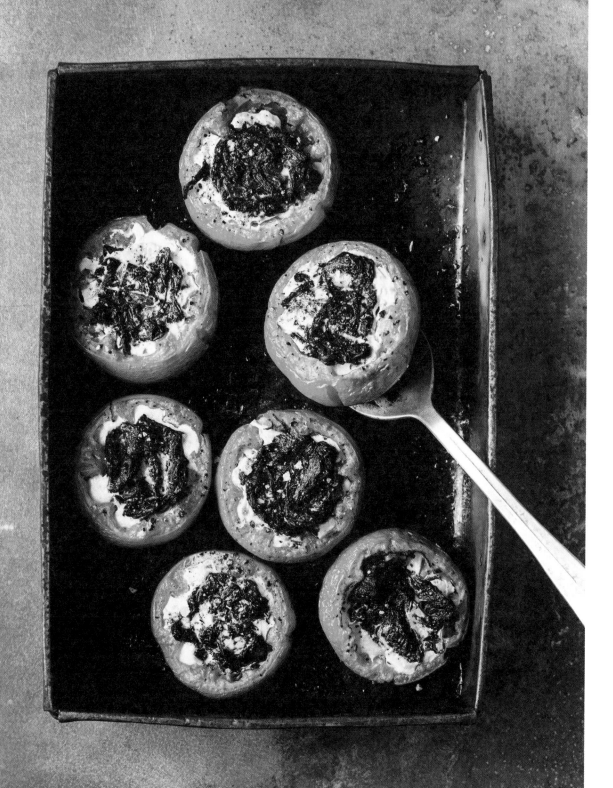

All-purpose mixed vegetable stir-fry

While interesting stir-fry combinations are great, I felt it was important here to include a really good all-round, side-dish stir-fry that can be served with almost anything – on top of some brown rice or quinoa, with meat, with fish, with a vegetarian main. This is one of those sides that is a staple fall-back recipe.

Serves: 2

1 tablespoon olive oil
2 cloves garlic, finely chopped
1 large red onion, peeled, halved
   and sliced
1 large red (bell) pepper, seeded and
   chopped into 1cm (½ inch) pieces
1 courgette (zucchini), sliced into rounds
2 teaspoons light soy sauce
2 teaspoons toasted sesame oil
1 teaspoon honey
1 teaspoon English mustard
½ teaspoon cornflour (cornstarch),
   dissolved in a little water

Heat the oil in a wok or wide pan. Add the garlic and onion and stir-fry for 2–3 minutes. Add the remaining vegetables and continue to stir-fry for around 5 minutes, until the vegetables are starting to soften.

Add the soy sauce, sesame oil, honey and mustard, and mix well. Add the dissolved cornflour (cornstarch) mixture and stir well on a high heat until a thick sauce forms.

Tuna pasta bake

Tuna pasta bake is one of those classic family dishes that just shouts comfort food, and this version gives the traditional one a bit of a facelift. In using brown pasta, we lower the glycaemic impact of the dish and increase the fibre, and the additional vegetables bring a load of extra micronutrients.

Serves: 2–3

300g (10½oz) wholewheat
   penne pasta
olive oil, for cooking
1 large red onion, finely chopped
3 cloves garlic, finely chopped
1 large courgette (zucchini), sliced
   into rounds

small bunch basil, roughly chopped
500g (1lb 2oz) passata (strained
   tomatoes)
2 x 160g (5oz) cans tuna, drained
3 handfuls baby spinach
100g (3½oz) goat cheese
sea salt
crisp green salad, to serve

Preheat the oven to 180°C/350°F/Gas mark 4.

Place the pasta in a pan, cover with boiling water and simmer as per packet instructions until soft to the bite. Drain and set aside.

While the pasta is cooking, heat a little oil in a frying pan, add the onion, garlic, courgette (zucchini) and a good pinch of salt and sauté for a few minutes until the onion is soft.

Add the basil and passata (strained tomatoes) and simmer for about 20 minutes, until the passata thickens into a rich sauce. Add the tuna and baby spinach, stir well and simmer for 2–3 minutes until the spinach has wilted.

Add the drained pasta to the sauce, mix well, then transfer to a deep oven dish. Crumble over the goat cheese and bake for 20 minutes. Serve with a crisp green salad.

Szechuan tofu and mangetout stir-fry

This is a lovely rich dish with a bit of zing – good for lunch. It could also be a vegetarian side, or a happy accompaniment to meat or poultry dishes.

Serves: 2

1 tablespoon olive oil
3 cloves garlic, finely chopped
2.5cm (1 inch) root ginger, peeled and
   cut into thin matchsticks
½ red chilli (chile), thinly sliced
   (seeds left in)
120g (4¼oz) mangetout (snow peas)
200g (7oz) firm tofu (bean curd), cubed
1 tablespoon tomato purée (paste)
2 teaspoons dark soy sauce
2 teaspoons apple cider vinegar
2 teaspoons honey

Heat the oil in a wok or wide pan. Throw in the garlic, ginger and chilli (chile) and stir-fry for about 1 minute. Add the mangetout (snow peas) and continue to stir-fry for 5–6 minutes.

Add the tofu (bean curd), tomato purée (paste), soy sauce, vinegar and honey, mix well and simmer for another 2–3 minutes before serving.

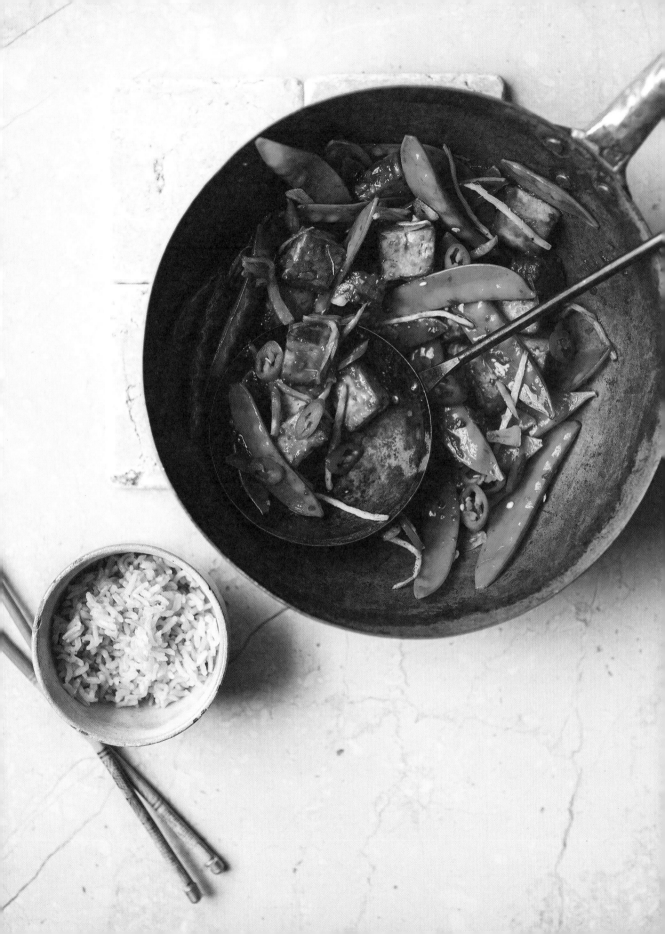

Wasabi salmon with courgette, carrot and sesame stir-fry

Salmon and wasabi are pretty much a match made in heaven. Being a sushi obsessive myself, I particularly love this pairing.

Serves: 2

2 teaspoons wasabi paste
2 teaspoons honey
2 teaspoons light soy sauce
2 salmon fillets
1 large carrot
1 large courgette (zucchini)
1 tablespoon olive oil
2 teaspoons toasted sesame oil
2 tablespoons sesame seeds

Preheat the oven to 180°C/350°F/Gas mark 4.

Mix the wasabi, honey, soy sauce, and 1 teaspoon water together to make a sauce.

Put the salmon on an oiled, foil-lined baking sheet and top with the sauce. Bake for 25 minutes.

Using a vegetable peeler, slice down the carrot and courgette (zucchini) to create ribbons. Do this for the whole carrot and courgette so as to make a type of pasta or noodle alternative.

Heat the olive oil in a pan or wok. Add the carrot and courgette and stir-fry until beginning to soften. Add the sesame oil and sesame seeds.

Serve each baked salmon fillet on top of the stir-fried courgette and carrot ribbons.

- STIR-FRYING
- FISH AND SEAFOOD
- ✕ PERFECT FOR DINNER

Kale and king prawn lemongrass stir-fry

This super-simple stir-fry goes brilliantly with noodles, quinoa, or rice.

Serves: 2

2 cloves garlic, finely chopped
2 large spring onions (scallions),
  sliced on the diagonal
2 lemongrass stalks, bashed with
  a rolling pin
olive oil, for frying
150g (5¼oz) cooked king prawns
  (shrimp)
3 handfuls curly kale, chopped
1 teaspoon dark soy sauce
Juice of ¼ lime

Sauté the garlic, spring onions (scallions), and bashed lemongrass in a little olive oil for 4–5 minutes until fragrant.

Add the king prawns (shrimp) and continue to sauté for another 2 minutes. Add the kale and sauté until wilted.

Add the soy sauce and lime juice and keep on the heat for another 1-2 minutes before serving.

Malay-style stir-fried rice noodles

I have been lucky enough to spend a good chunk of time in Malaysia, and the food in that country is off-the-chart amazing: a melting pot of Thai, Chinese, Indian, French and Portuguese influences, all shook up. The result is flavoursome, spiced, rich, exciting food. This is a complete dish in itself, although you could have some garlicky greens alongside if you like.

Serves: 2

2 bundles rice noodles
1 tablespoon olive oil
2 cloves garlic, finely chopped
1 red chilli (chile), finely chopped
   (seeds left in)
1 large red onion, peeled,
   halved and sliced
2 lemongrass stalks, bashed
   with a rolling pin

1 star anise
handful curly kale, shredded
60g (2oz) shiitake mushrooms, sliced
sea salt

For the sauce
1½ tablespoons crunchy peanut butter
2 teaspoons light soy sauce
2 teaspoons honey

Place the rice noodles in a heatproof bowl and cover with just-boiled water. Allow to soften for 5–10 minutes, then drain and set aside.

Heat the oil in a wok or wide pan. Throw in the garlic, chilli (chile), red onion, lemongrass and star anise, along with a pinch of salt, and stir-fry until the onion has softened and the lemongrass and star anise are becoming fragrant. Add the kale and mushrooms and stir-fry for 2–3 minutes until the mushrooms and vegetables have softened.

Mix the peanut butter, soy sauce, honey and 2 tablespoons water together to make a sauce.

Add the noodles to the vegetables and toss well, then add the sauce and toss again. Simmer for a couple of minutes and add a little salt if needed.

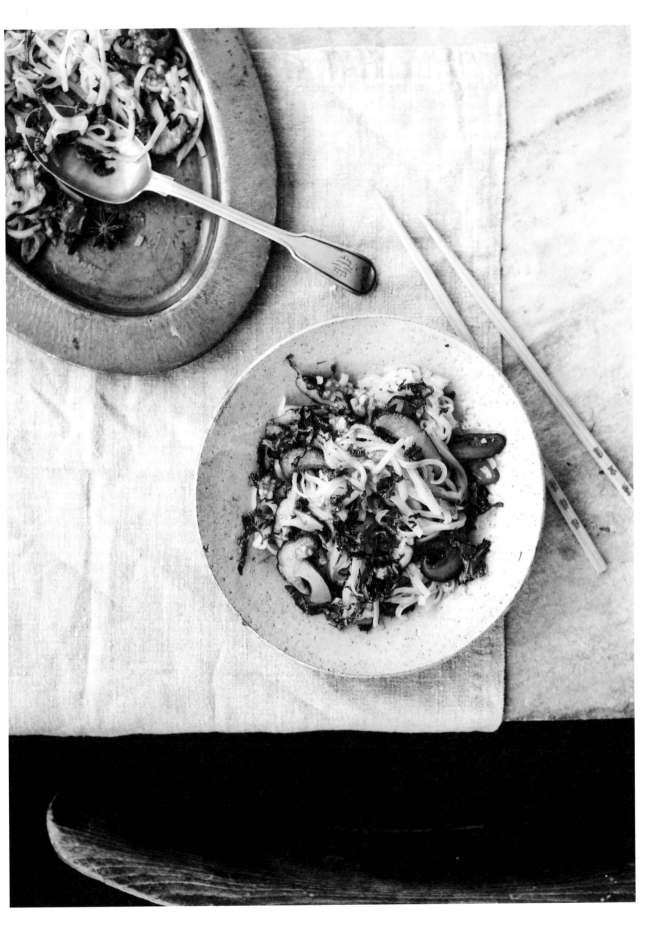

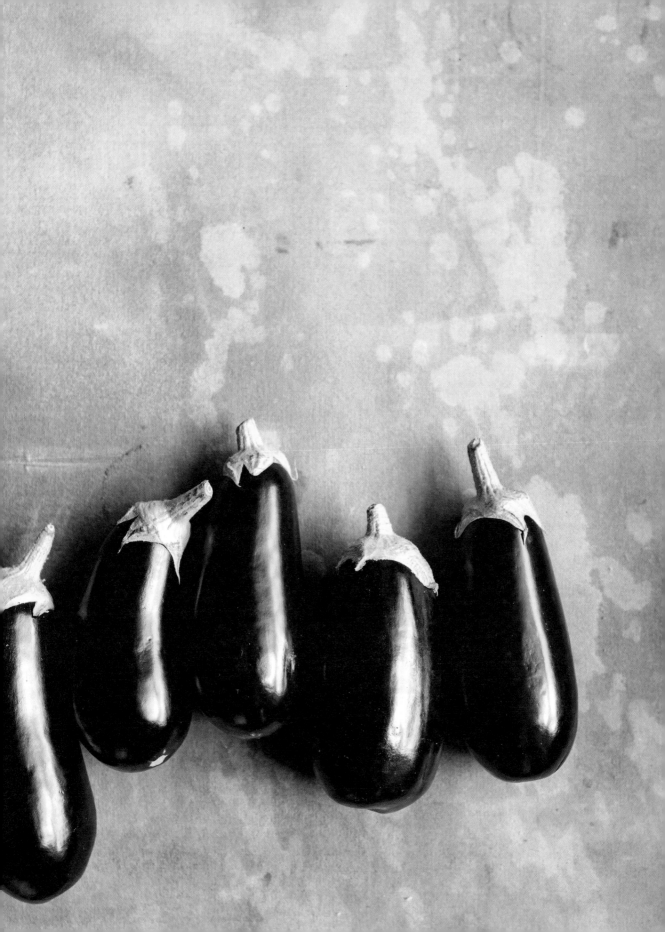

Miso aubergine

Asian fusion restaurants are becoming ultra-popular in our cities now, and one thing that has crept on to many a menu, much to my glee, is miso aubergine (eggplant). This amazing side dish is a little piece of heaven and one of my all-time favourites.

Serves: 2

1 tablespoon olive oil
1 large aubergine (eggplant), diced
2 teaspoons miso paste
1 teaspoon sesame oil
1 teaspoon sesame seeds

Heat the oil in a wok or wide pan. Throw in the diced aubergine (eggplant) and stir-fry for around 6 minutes or so until soft and beginning to turn golden.

Add the miso paste and sesame oil and mix well. Add the sesame seeds before serving.

Sweet potato boats

A healthier twist on the classic potato boats, these are great just served with a salad, or can be a substantial side dish to chicken or red meat. Using sweet potato instead of regular potato gives you a lower glycaemic impact, and also buckets of beta carotene from the bright orange flesh. The fats in the goat cheese increase beta-carotene absorption.

Serves: 2

1 large sweet potato, halved lengthways
150g (5¼oz) soft, fresh goat cheese
2 teaspoons English mustard
small handful curly parsley, roughly
   chopped
sea salt and black pepper

Preheat the oven to 200°C/400°F/Gas mark 6.

Using a sharp knife, score the exposed flesh of the sweet potato halves, about 2.5cm (1 inch) deep, and place them flesh side down on a baking sheet. Bake for around 20 minutes, then check by giving one a gentle squeeze: if it gives under very little pressure, they are done. If not, continue to bake until softened.

Remove from the oven and, when just cool enough to handle, scoop the flesh out into a bowl, leaving the empty skins on the baking sheet ready to be refilled. Add the goat cheese, mustard, parsley and some salt and pepper to the sweet potato flesh and mash well to ensure the ingredients are all thoroughly mixed.

Spoon the mixture back in to the empty skins and return to the oven for around 15 minutes, just long enough for a gentle golden crust to form.

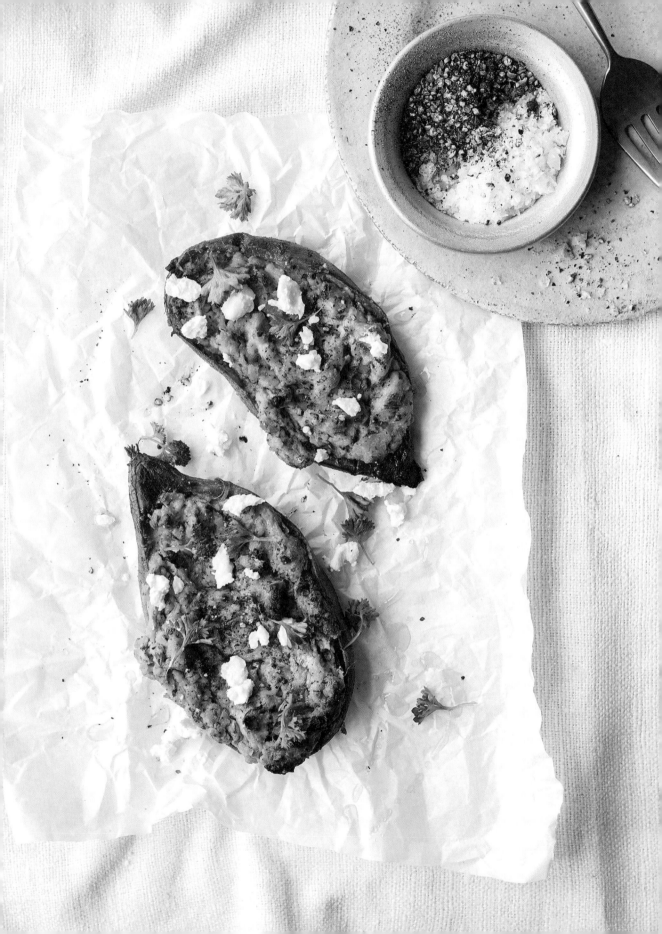

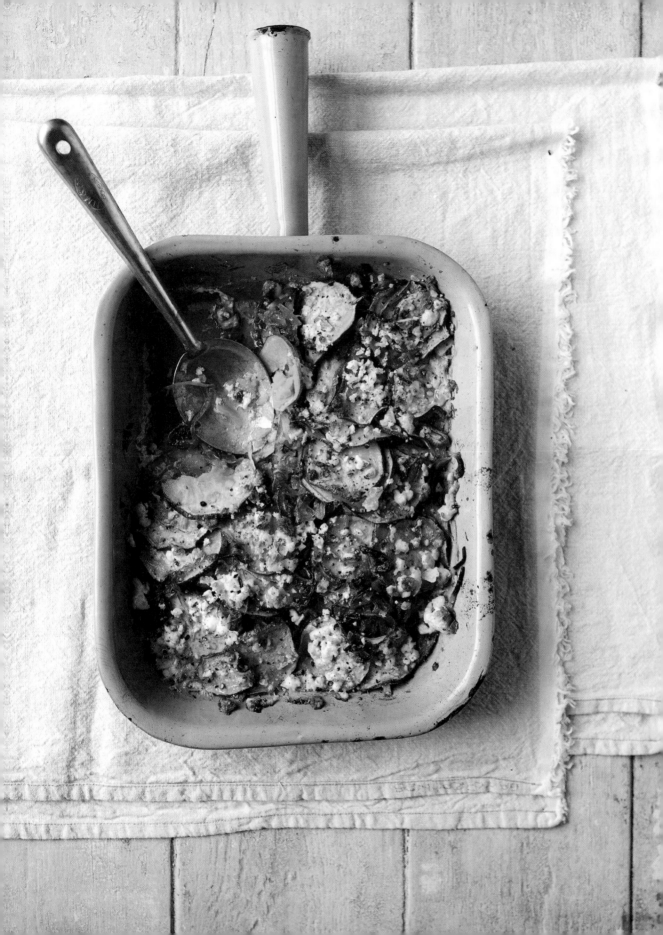

Celeriac and sweet potato gratin

This is a healthier version of the typical potato gratin, but is still just as comforting. It is great served with oily fish, or with a nice dense side salad.

Serves: 2

olive oil, for cooking
1 large red onion, finely chopped
250ml (scant 1 cup) milk
2 good sprigs thyme
2 cloves garlic, finely chopped
1 teaspoon vegetable bouillon powder
225g (8oz) celeriac, peeled and sliced
500g (1lb 2oz) sweet potato, sliced
   (skin left on)
80g (2¾oz) feta cheese
sea salt

Preheat the oven to 180°C/350°F/Gas mark 4.

Heat a little oil in a frying pan, add the onion and a good pinch of salt and sauté until softened.

Put the milk in a saucepan with the thyme, garlic and bouillon powder and simmer gently for a minute or two, just to the point where the milk starts to boil, stirring almost constantly. Remove from the heat.

Line the base of a large baking dish with a layer of celeriac slices, then sweet potato slices. Repeat this until half of the sweet potato and celeriac have been used. Pour in half the milk mixture and add the sautéed onions on top, then begin layering again, so that the onions end up sandwiched in the middle. Pour over the remaining milk mixture.

Crumble the feta cheese over the top, then bake for around 1½ hours, until the top is golden and all the layers are soft; a fork or skewer pushed through should go in easily.

Red lentil, butternut squash and fennel casserole

This is a super-easy, warming and hearty dish. It's great served with fish, or on its own in a massive bowl on a cold night.

Serves: 2

180g (1 cup) red lentils
¼ butternut squash, diced (skin left on)
½ fennel bulb, sliced lengthways
½ red onion, sliced
about 500ml (generous 2 cups)
   vegetable stock

Preheat the oven to 180°C/350°F/Gas mark 4.

Place the lentils, squash, fennel and onion in a casserole dish. Pour the stock over and bake in the oven for about 1 hour, checking once or twice and stirring if necessary – you are aiming for a texture similar to porridge from the lentils breaking down, with the vegetables nice and soft, so add more vegetable stock or water if it seems too thick.

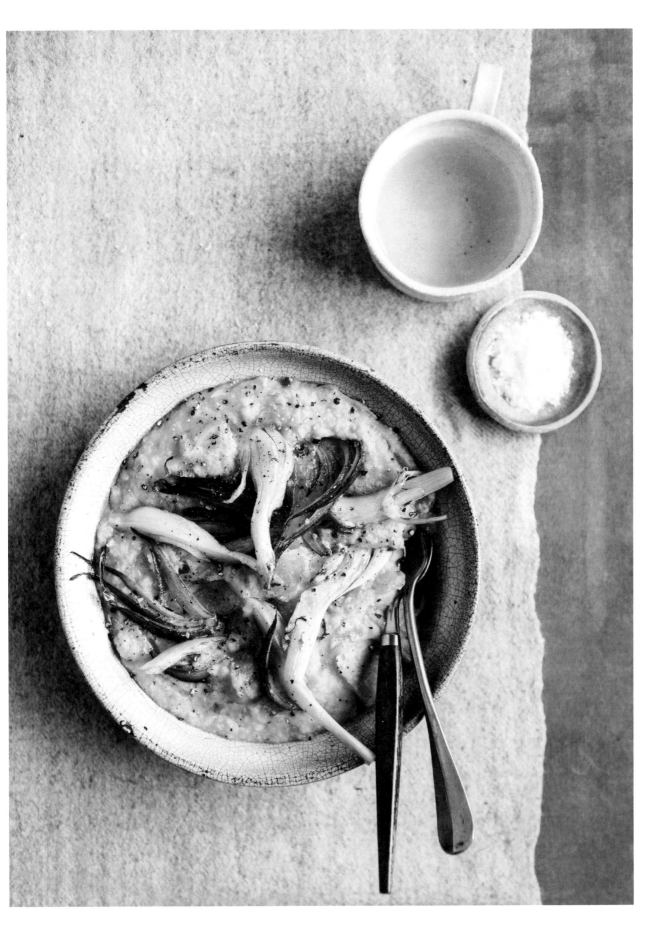

Sweet potato-topped vegetarian cottage pie

This is a real winter favourite in Pinnock Towers! I have made this a veggie one as it's a recipe that works very well, but you can absolutely use the traditional minced (ground) beef if you like. The sweet potato topping is lower GI than regular potato, plus the bright orange flesh is rich in beta carotene, which is a potent antioxidant.

Serves: 4

900g (just under 2lb) sweet potato (peeling is optional), cut into chunks
olive oil, for cooking
1 large red onion, finely chopped
2 cloves garlic, finely chopped
2 large carrots, cut into small dice

1 x 400g (14oz) can green lentils, drained
1 x 400g (14oz) can chopped tomatoes
2 sprigs thyme
½ teaspoon ground cinnamon
1 teaspoon vegetable bouillon powder
sea salt

Preheat the oven to 180°C/350°F/Gas mark 4.

Place the chopped sweet potato in a saucepan, cover with boiling water and simmer until soft. Drain, mash well and set aside.

While the sweet potato is cooking, heat a little oil in a large saucepan, add the onion, garlic, carrots and a good pinch of salt, and sauté until the onion has softened.

Add the lentils, tomatoes, thyme, cinnamon and bouillon powder, and simmer for around 20 minutes, until the tomatoes have reduced right down to create a thick sauce with the lentils.

Transfer to a deep baking dish, top with the mashed sweet potato and bake in the oven for around 20 minutes.

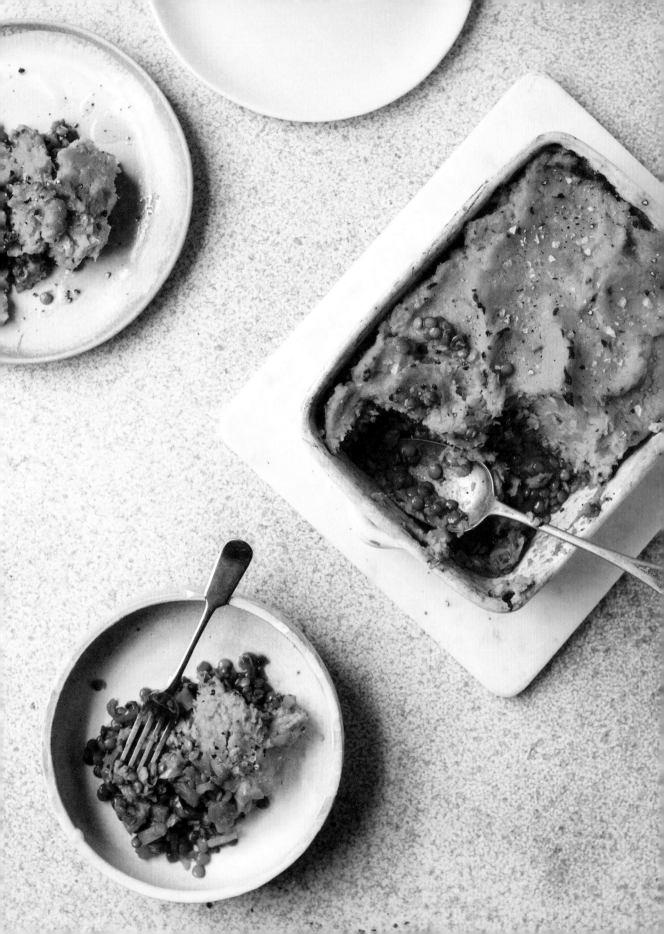

Citrus and thyme-roasted Mediterranean vegetables

This is a lovely zingy accompaniment to all manner of dishes. Great with fish or chicken, or even served cold in a salad with some goat cheese.

Serves: 2–3

1 large red onion, peeled,
  halved and sliced
1 large courgette (zucchini),
  sliced into rounds
2 red (bell) peppers, seeded
  and sliced lengthways
4–6 chestnut (cremini) mushrooms,
  sliced
1 tablespoon olive oil
finely grated zest of 1 lemon and
  juice of ½
finely grated zest of 1 lime and juice of ½
3 sprigs thyme
sea salt and black pepper

Preheat the oven to 200°C/400°F/Gas mark 6.

Place all the sliced vegetables in a roasting tray. Drizzle the olive oil and the lemon and lime juice over the vegetables and toss well.

Add the lemon and lime zest. Remove the thyme leaves from their stalks by pinching the base of the stalks between thumb and forefinger and, using the nails of the thumb and forefinger, pull upwards along the stalk to remove the leaves. Add the leaves to the vegetables, along with some salt and pepper, and toss again.

Roast for 20–25 minutes, stirring occasionally.

Mushroom-stuffed chicken breast

This is a lovely little dish that looks awesome when served carefully sliced. I make all manner of variations of this as a Sunday lunch, with the usual trimmings. It can be served with salad, roasted vegetables... or any sides you fancy.

Serves: 2

olive oil, for cooking
1 clove garlic, finely chopped
small sprig rosemary
10 button mushrooms, roughly
   chopped
2 teaspoons full-fat cream cheese
2 large skinless, boneless chicken
   breasts
4 slices smoked bacon
sea salt and black pepper

Preheat the oven to 180°C/350°F/Gas mark 4.

Heat a little oil in a frying pan, add the garlic, rosemary sprig and a pinch of salt and sauté for 2–3 minutes. Add the mushrooms and cook until they are soft and dark in colour.

Discard the rosemary sprig. Add the cream cheese and mix well. Using a potato masher, mash the mixture to create a coarse-pâté texture. Taste and adjust the seasoning if necessary.

Slice along the side of each chicken breast to make a pocket. Stuff each pocket with the mushroom mixture, then wrap 2 bacon slices around each chicken breast to hold it together and prevent the mushroom stuffing from leaking out. Place on a baking sheet and bake for 20–25 minutes, until cooked through.

● MEAT AND POULTRY
● ROASTING AND BAKING
✗ PERFECT FOR A FAMILY LUNCH

Chinese-style roast chicken

This is an amazing flavoursome twist on everyday roast chicken. As it needs to be left overnight, it is a great one to prep on Saturday afternoon for a Sunday roast.

Serves: 4

1 medium chicken

For the marinade
3 tablespoons light soy sauce
1½ teaspoons runny honey
½ teaspoon Chinese five-spice powder
1 teaspoon toasted sesame oil
¼ teaspoon sea salt

For the glaze
1 tablespoon olive oil
½ teaspoon toasted sesame oil
1 teaspoon honey

Mix all the marinade ingredients together.

Place the chicken in a large plastic food bag (with a seal). Pour the marinade into the bag, seal and then shake and/or rotate the bag to make sure the chicken is covered in the marinade. Place in the fridge overnight, rotating or shaking it every few hours to ensure that the chicken gets well marinated and that the marinade doesn't just accumulate in one area.

When ready to cook, preheat the oven to 200°C/400°F/Gas mark 6. Remove the chicken from the bag, place in a roasting tin and roast for 1 hour, then remove from the oven. Mix the glaze ingredients together, then brush the glaze all over the chicken and roast for another 25 minutes (or the remaining cooking time, calculated by weight).

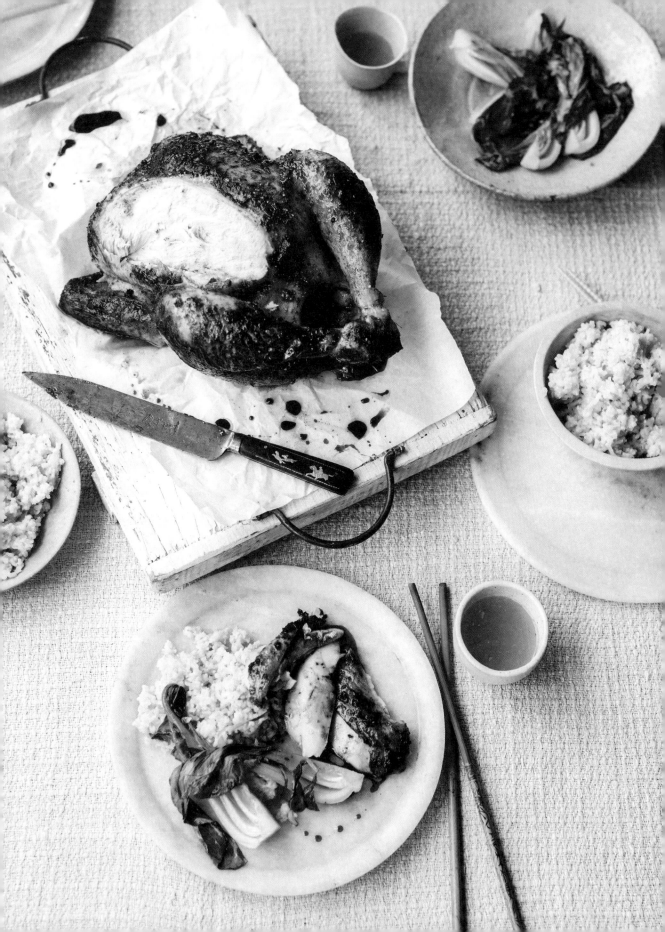

Red-curry chicken burgers with apple ginger slaw

These are an awesome lunch or barbecue option. Packed with flavour, the apple ginger slaw takes it to another level, not to mention adding in more potent nutrients.

Serves: 2–3

2 skinless, boneless chicken breasts, roughly chopped
2 tablespoons Thai red curry paste
1 large clove garlic, finely chopped
¼ red onion, finely chopped
small bunch coriander (cilantro), roughly chopped
olive oil, for frying
Little Gem (Bibb) lettuce leaves, to serve
sea salt

For the slaw

1 Cox apple, cored and cut into matchsticks
2.5cm (1 inch) root ginger, peeled and cut into matchsticks
½ teaspoon caraway seeds
1 tablespoon mayonnaise
juice of ¼ lime

Place the chicken breast, curry paste, garlic, onion, coriander (cilantro) and a generous pinch of salt in a food processor, and process until minced (ground). Form into small burger patties and set aside.

Combine the slaw ingredients, with a pinch of salt added, and mix well.

Heat a little oil in a frying pan until hot, add the burgers and pan-fry for 4–5 minutes on each side, until golden brown and cooked through. Place each burger on a lettuce leaf, top with the slaw and serve with a side salad.

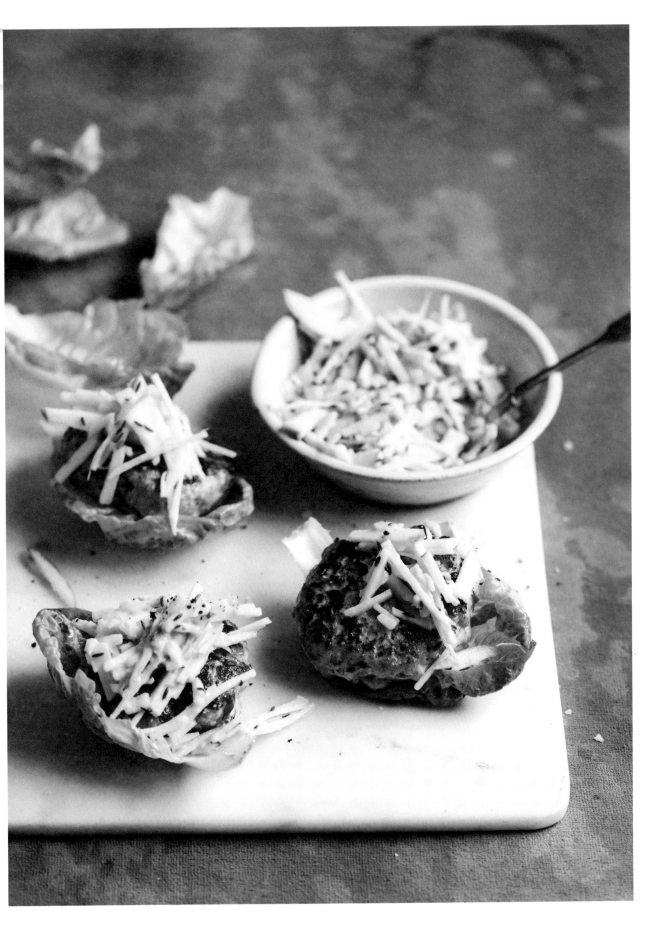

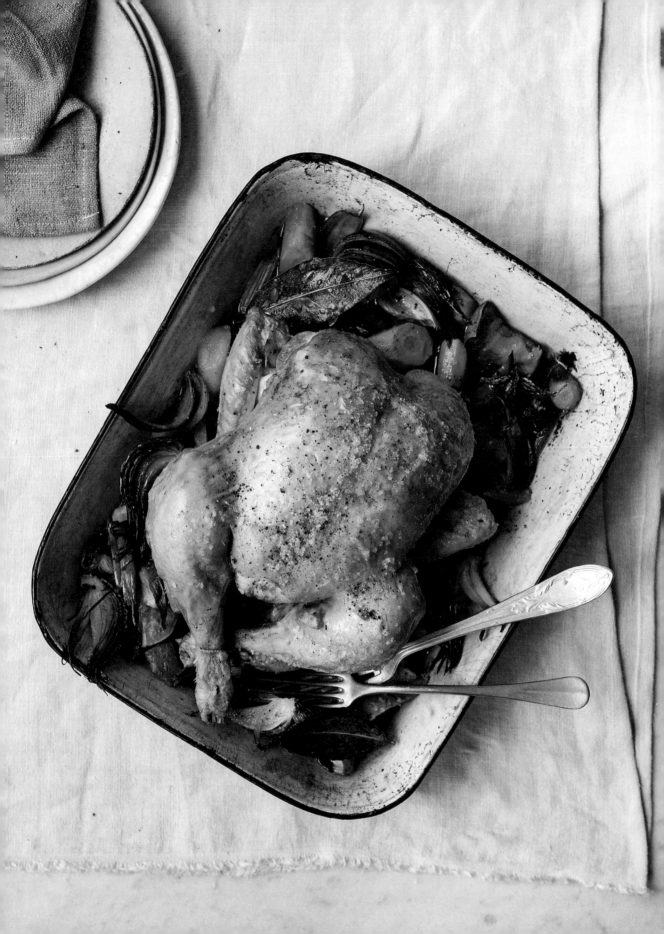

Chicken tray bake

This is a similar basis from which I make my Sunday roasts, except then I use the vegetables in the tray and the meat juices to make a separate, rich gravy. Here the meat juices flow into the vegetables and everything cooks down together to make a serious bit of comfort food.

Serves: 3–4

1 large sweet potato, diced
1 red onion, peeled, halved and sliced
   lengthways
2 celery stalks, sliced
2 carrots, sliced
4 cloves garlic, 2 left whole, unpeeled
   and smashed; 2 finely sliced
2 bay leaves
1 cinnamon stick
1 small chicken
sea salt and black pepper

Preheat the oven to 200°C/400°F/Gas mark 6.

Spread the vegetables out in a deep roasting tray, with the 2 whole, smashed garlic cloves (reserve the sliced garlic) bay leaves and cinnamon.

Place the chicken on top of the vegetables. Using a knife, cut small incisions into the chicken flesh and push individual slices of garlic into the incisions.

Sprinkle with salt and pepper and roast for around 1 hour. Remove from the oven and transfer the chicken to a clean, separate roasting tray. Return the chicken to the oven for a further 20 minutes, until cooked.

Place the tray with the roasted vegetables on the hob (stove top). Add 200ml (generous ¾ cup) water, turn up the heat and simmer for 2–3 minutes so that all the meat juices and flavours mix together with the water to make a thick sauce that will cling to the roasted vegetables. Carve the chicken and serve with the roasted vegetables.

Stuffed chicken breasts

This is a great-looking dish, gently cut into slices to reveal its vibrant centre. Serve with some roasted root vegetables or a simple salad.

Serves: 1

2 handfuls baby spinach
1 tablespoon full-fat cream cheese
small sprig dill, roughly chopped
1 large skinless, boneless chicken breast
sea salt and cracked black pepper

Put the spinach into a small bowl, place the bowl in the steamer and steam for 2–3 minutes until it wilts. Remove the spinach, squeeze to remove as much moisture as possible, then cut into shreds with a knife and put into the (dried out) bowl. Add the cream cheese, dill and some salt and pepper, and mix well.

Cut a slice along the side of the chicken breast but not all the way through, to create a pocket. Stuff the spinach mixture into the pocket, then seal the breast closed using cocktail sticks (toothpicks). Place the stuffed breast on a small plate and place in a steamer. Steam for 20 minutes.

Remove the cocktail sticks and allow to cool slightly before gently slicing.

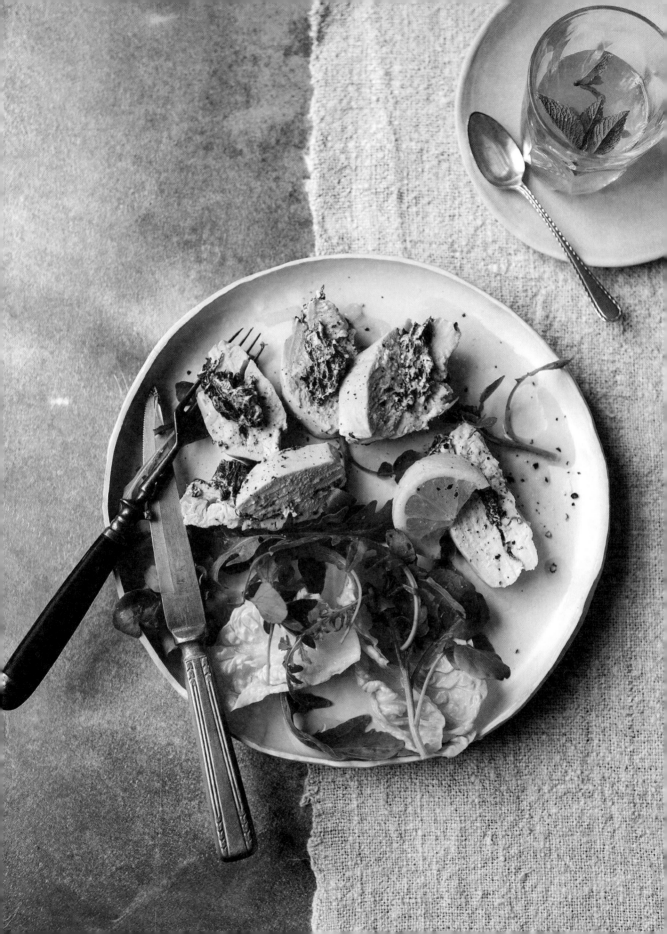

Sticky chilli chicken and greens

This is a truly comforting dish. While there is a bit of honey used, which can send the sugar content up, if you serve it with some brown rice, the fibre will slow down its release so it shouldn't cause major blood sugar issues.

Serves: 2

olive oil, for cooking
2 skinless, boneless chicken
   breasts, diced
2 handfuls curly kale, chopped
1 tablespoon honey
2 teaspoons light soy sauce
1 teaspoon toasted sesame oil
3 cloves garlic, finely chopped
1 red chilli (chile), finely chopped

Heat a little olive oil in a wok or large saucepan. Add the chicken and stir-fry for about 5–6 minutes, until the chicken is cooked through. Add the kale and cook until softened.

Add the honey, soy sauce, sesame oil, garlic and chilli (chile), and continue to stir-fry until the honey has caramelized and the sauce is a sticky golden colour.

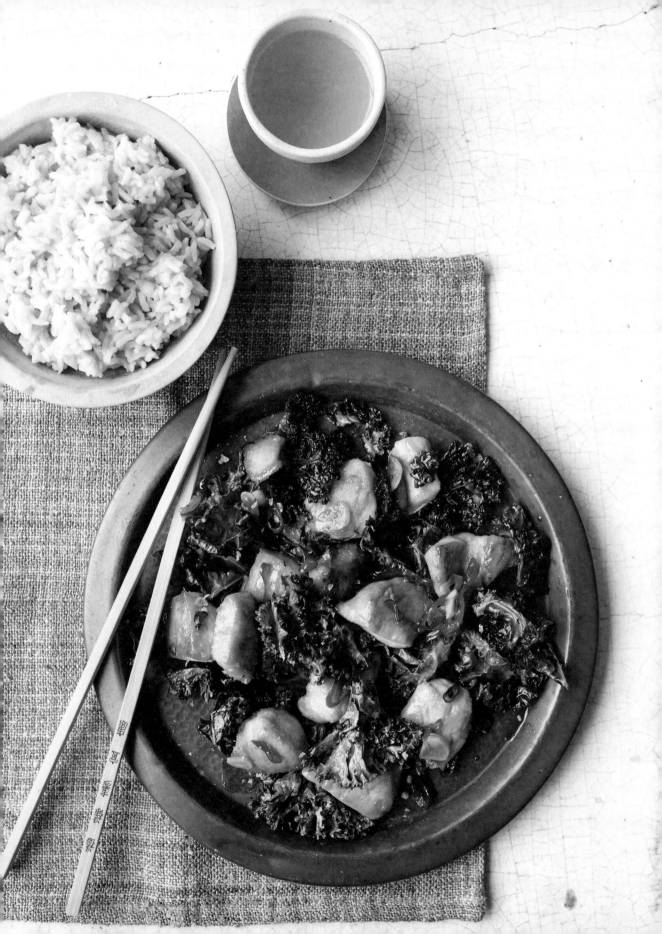

Herbed turkey meatballs with courgetti pomodoro

Unless you have been living in a parallel universe, chances are you will have seen spiralizers that make "noodles" out of vegetables for a great pasta alternative. There are hundreds of recipes for courgette (zucchini) or carrot noodles out there, so this is the only one I'm going to give you, just to demonstrate the possibilities. You don't even need a spiralizer – supermarkets now have ready-prepared courgette noodles if you're really short on time.

Serves: 4

1 large courgette (zucchini)

For the meatballs
500g (1lb 2oz) minced (ground) turkey
2 cloves garlic, finely chopped
½ red onion, finely chopped
8–10g (⅓oz) flat-leaf parsley, finely chopped
8–10g (⅓oz) basil leaves, finely chopped, plus extra to serve
1 egg

For the sauce
olive oil, for cooking
½ red onion, finely chopped
2 cloves garlic, finely chopped
400g (14oz) passata (strained tomatoes)
1 teaspoon dried mixed herbs
sea salt

Begin by making the sauce. Heat a little oil in a pan, add the onion, garlic and a good pinch of salt and sauté until the onion has softened. Add the passata (strained tomatoes) and mixed herbs and simmer for 25 minutes or so. You are aiming for a thick, rich sauce.

Mix the meatball ingredients together well and roll into balls. Add the meatballs to the sauce and simmer for 20 minutes, to cook through.

Using a spiralizer, make noodles from the courgette (zucchini). Place the noodles in the centre of a plate and top with the meatballs, sauce and basil to garnish.

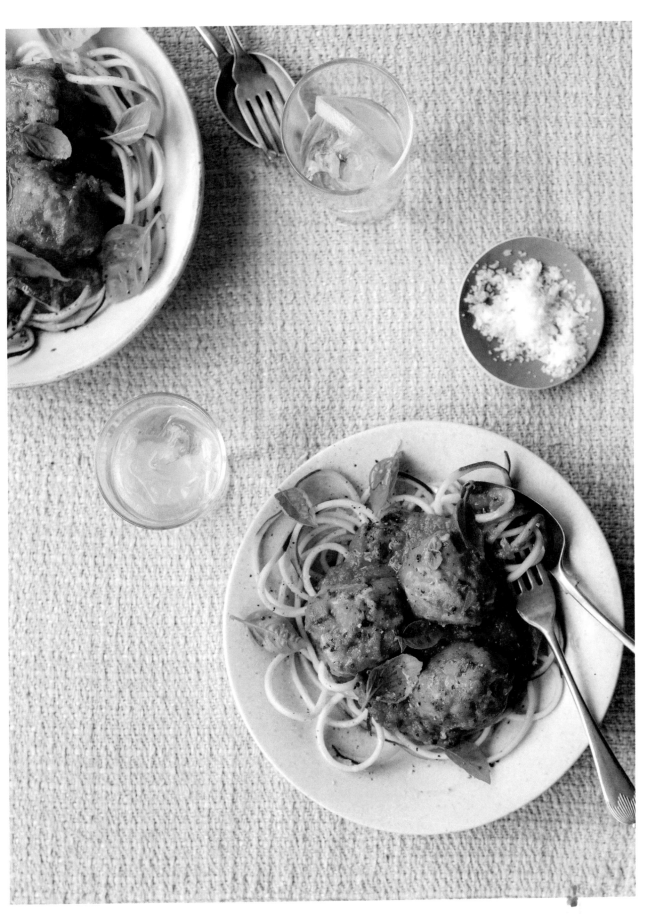

- ● MEAT AND POULTRY
- ● GOOD FATS
- ✗ PERFECT FOR DINNER

Nutty Southeast Asian turkey hotpot

This is such a tasty little number. Rich, well spiced, fragrant, creamy, it works well with chicken and duck, too. It's an excellent way of using up leftovers.

Serves: 2

½ tablespoon coconut oil
1 red onion, finely chopped
3 cloves garlic, finely chopped
1 small green chilli (chile), finely chopped
2 lemongrass stalks, bashed with a
   rolling pin
400ml (1¾ cups) coconut milk
1 heaped tablespoon crunchy
   peanut butter
½ teaspoon ground turmeric
2 turkey breast fillets, diced
large handful spinach
juice of ½ lime
sea salt or pink crystal salt

Melt the coconut oil in a pan, add the onion, garlic, chilli (chile), lemongrass and a generous pinch of salt, and sauté until the onion is nice and soft.

Add the coconut milk, stir in the peanut butter and turmeric, and simmer for around 10 minutes until the sauce thickens and the flavour of the lemongrass is really starting to come through.

Add the diced turkey and continue to simmer for at least 10 minutes to ensure the meat is fully cooked. Add the spinach and stir until it wilts. Squeeze in the lime juice, check the seasoning and serve.

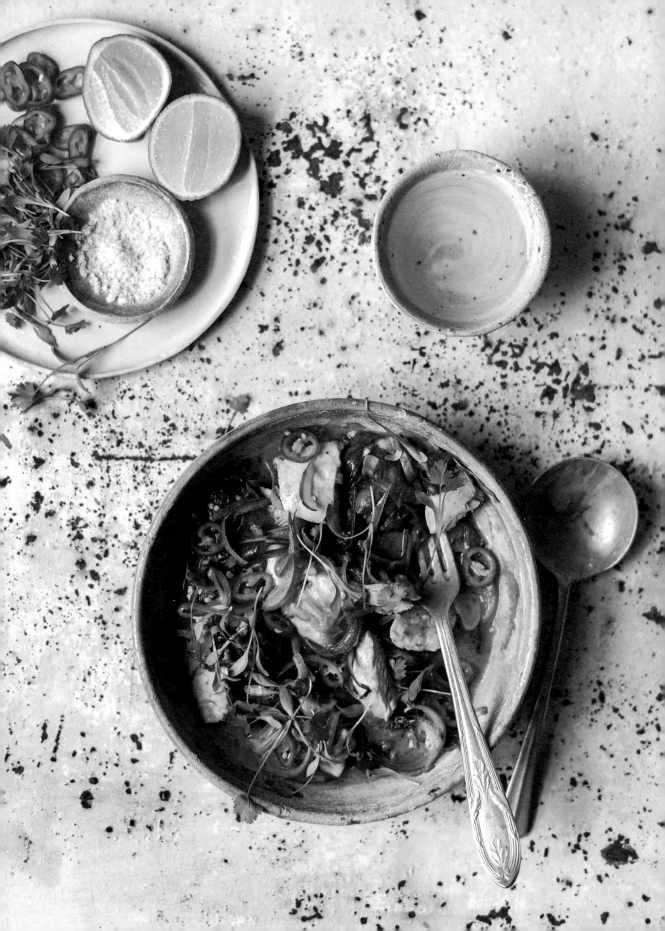

Seared beef and pomegranate salad

This is a lovely, fresh, zingy summer salad. I prefer the steak seared, but feel free to cook it to well done, if you prefer.

Serves: 2

2 large handfuls mixed salad leaves
4–5 cherry tomatoes, halved
1 sirloin steak
½ pomegranate

For the dressing
2 teaspoons pomegranate molasses
1 tablespoon extra virgin olive oil
½ clove garlic, finely chopped
pinch sea salt

Combine the salad leaves and tomatoes on a serving plate.

Place a frying pan over a high heat and, when hot, place the steak in it. Fry on each side for 1–2 minutes (or longer if you prefer it well done). Remove to a board and let it rest for a couple of minutes before slicing it into thin strips.

Holding the halved pomegranate over the plate of salad, hit the rounded side with a wooden spoon to release and sprinkle the seeds over the leaves. Add the steak slices to the salad.

Mix the dressing ingredients together and whisk well before dressing the salad to serve.

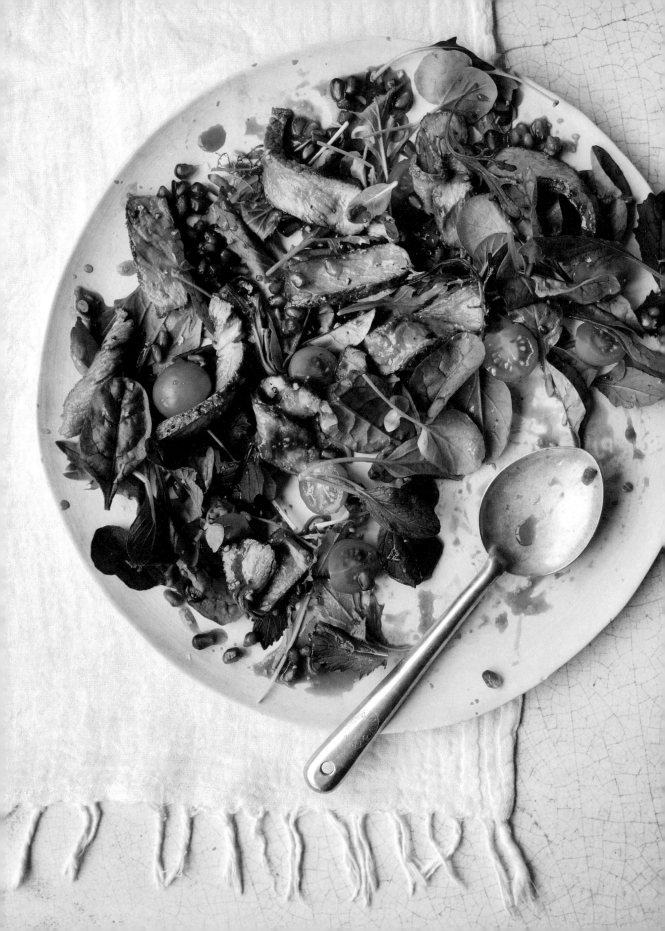

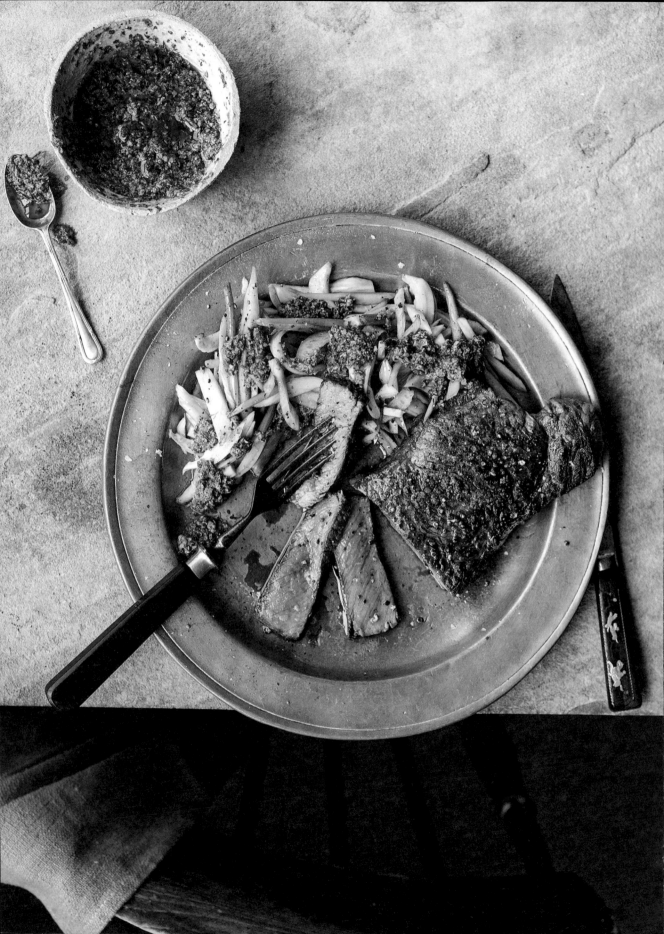

Steak with salsa verde and shredded fennel salad

I absolutely love this dish. Fresh, vibrant, crisp. Amazing stuff.

Serves: 1

15g (½oz) flat-leaf parsley
50g (1¾oz) capers
1 clove garlic
3 tablespoons olive oil
1 large fennel bulb
1 teaspoon balsamic vinegar
1 sirloin steak
sea salt and black pepper

For the salsa verde, place the parsley, capers, garlic and 2 tablespoons of the oil in a small food processor and process to a smooth green sauce. Set aside.

Slice the fennel thinly lengthways. Lay the slices flat and slice again lengthways to create long, thin shards.

Mix the balsamic vinegar, remaining tablespoon of olive oil and some salt and pepper together. Dress the shredded fennel with this vinaigrette and toss well.

Place a frying pan over a high heat and, when hot, place the steak in it. Fry on each side for 1–2 minutes (or longer if you prefer it well done). Place a pile of the fennel salad in the centre of a plate and top with the steak. Drizzle the salsa verde generously over the top.

Beef moussaka with yogurt "béchamel"

This is a great twist on the classic moussaka, with the yogurt topping creating a lighter dish.

Serves: 2–3

2 aubergines (eggplants), thinly sliced
olive oil, for cooking
1 large red onion, finely chopped
2 cloves garlic, finely chopped
500g (1lb 2oz) minced (ground) beef
400g (14oz) passata (strained
  tomatoes)
2 teaspoons ground cinnamon

1 teaspoon dried mixed herbs
sea salt and black pepper

For the topping
1 teaspoon cornflour (cornstarch)
300g (10½oz) Greek yogurt
2 eggs
pinch freshly grated nutmeg (optional)
50g (¾ cup) freshly grated Parmesan cheese

Preheat the oven to 180°C/350°F/Gas mark 4. Spread the aubergine (eggplant) slices out on a baking sheet in a single layer. Brush with a little olive oil and bake for about 20–25 minutes until nice and soft.

Heat a little oil in a pan, add the onion, garlic and a good pinch of salt and sauté until the onion has softened. Add the beef and cook until it changes colour. Add the passata (strained tomatoes) and half the cinnamon and simmer until the passata has reduced and you have a thick sauce. Add the dried herbs and remaining cinnamon, then taste and adjust the seasoning if necessary. Spoon a thin layer of the meat sauce into an ovenproof dish, about 28 x 20cm (11 x 8 inches) and 6cm (2½ inches) deep. Add a layer of aubergine slices on top, then another layer of meat sauce, repeating until both ingredients are used up.

Make the topping by mixing the cornflour (cornstarch) into a small amount of the yogurt, until smooth. Add the remaining yogurt, then whisk the eggs into the mixture. Add some salt, pepper and nutmeg, if you like, then add the Parmesan and mix well. Spoon the topping over the meat mixture and bake for 45–50 minutes, until the topping has set and is turning golden.

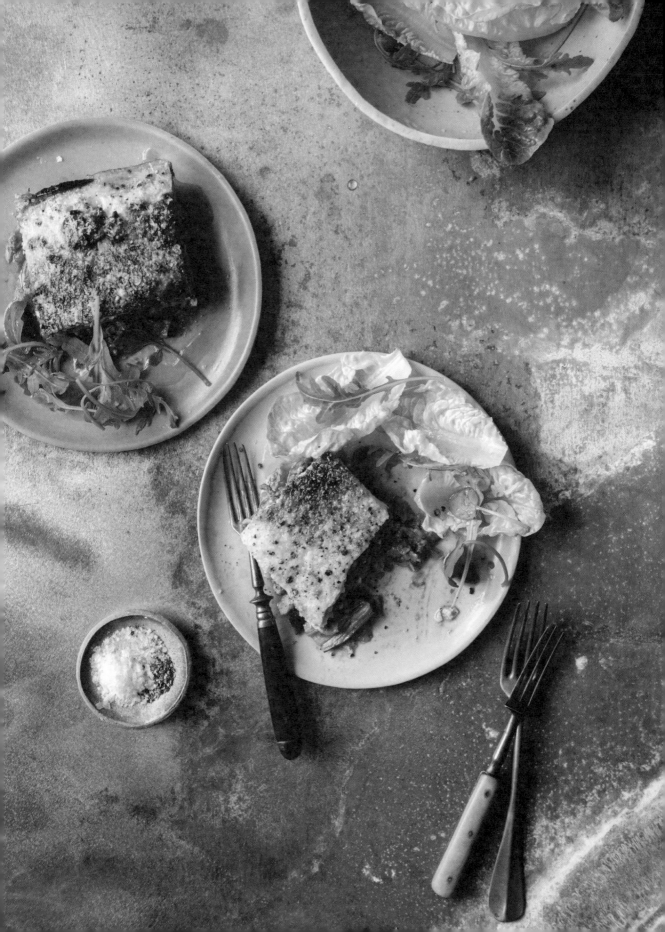

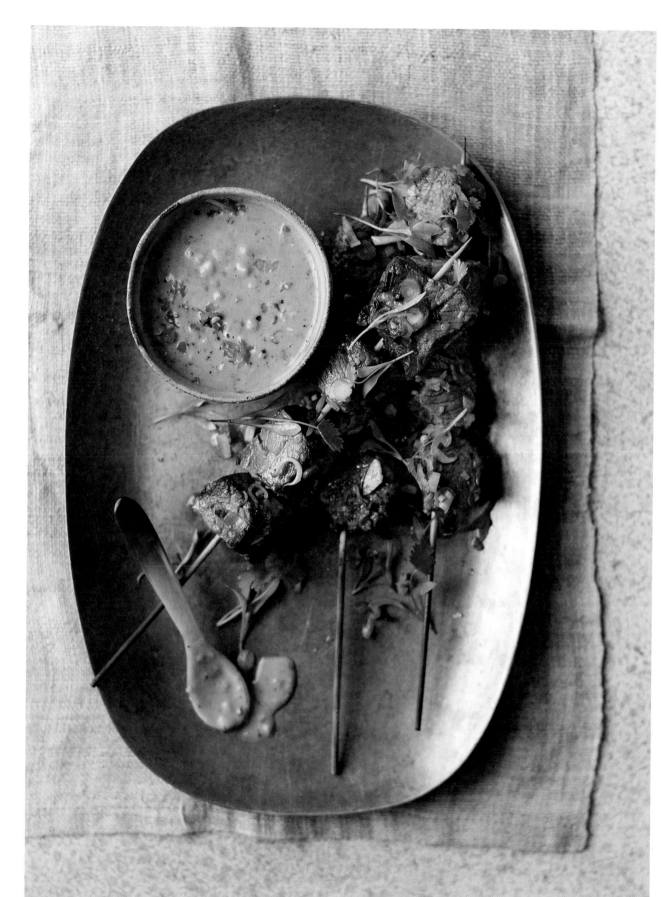

● MEAT AND POULTRY
● GOOD FATS
✗ PERFECT FOR DINNER

Beef satay

Having spent some time out in Malaysia, I soon became obsessed with satay. Delicious stuff. A really simple dish to make, but packed with flavour. As well as tasting great, it is seriously nutrient-dense: iron, zinc, B vitamins, magnesium… indulgent health!

Serves: 2

1 large sirloin steak, trimmed
  and diced

For the marinade
juice of ½ lime
1 lemongrass stalk, very finely
  chopped
1 clove garlic, finely chopped
2 teaspoons light soy sauce
¼ teaspoon ground turmeric

For the dipping sauce
1 heaped tablespoon peanut butter
½ lemongrass stalk, very finely chopped
1 clove garlic, finely chopped
1 small red chilli (chile), finely chopped
¼ teaspoon Chinese five-spice powder
2 teaspoons light soy sauce
3 tablespoons coconut milk

Mix all the marinade ingredients together in a bowl. Add the steak and leave to marinate in the fridge for at least 3–4 hours, ideally overnight.

When ready to cook, combine all the dipping sauce ingredients with 1 tablespoon water and mix well. (You may find that mixing the peanut butter and spices together first and adding the liquids a little at a time, mixing well between additions, will give you a better texture.) Set aside.

Remove the beef from the marinade and thread the chunks onto some skewers.

Line a baking sheet with foil and lay the beef skewers on it. Cook under a hot grill (broiler) for 15 minutes, turning regularly. Serve with the dipping sauce.

Roast pork with apple and fennel purée

This is one of my favourite Sunday lunches ever. The purée is an amazing twist on the traditional apple sauce, and the flavours work so beautifully together. I wouldn't have this every day, but it's a great example of how you can have the traditional favourites and do your health some favours at the same time.

Serves: 2–3

2 apples, cored and cut into wedges
1 large fennel bulb, sliced
1.3kg (2lb 14oz) pork belly roasting joint
olive oil, for drizzling
150g (5¼oz) purple sprouting broccoli
½ red chilli (chile), thinly sliced (optional)
sea salt

Preheat the oven to 180°C/350°F/Gas mark 4. Put the apple wedges and fennel in a roasting dish and rub lightly in olive oil. Roast for 30 minutes, or until soft and turning golden at the edges, and when they will squash easily when squeezed. Remove and set aside, and increase the oven temperature to 220°C/425°F/Gas mark 7.

If the pork skin is not already scored, score it at regular intervals, using a sharp knife. Drizzle a small amount of olive oil over the scored skin, along with a generous pinch of salt, and rub into the scores. Place in a roasting tray and roast at the top of the oven for 15 minutes, until the skin starts to blister and turn golden. Reduce the oven temperature to 180°C/350°F/Gas mark 4 and roast for another 2–2½ hours, checking the crackling regularly: crispy is perfect, burnt is bad. While the pork is roasting, place the roasted apple and fennel in a food processor with 2–3 teaspoons water, and process to a smooth purée. Alternatively, you can leave the apple and fennel whole if you prefer.

When the pork is almost done, steam the broccoli for 5–6 minutes, until just tender, adding a little chilli if you like. Serve with the purée, pork and crackling.

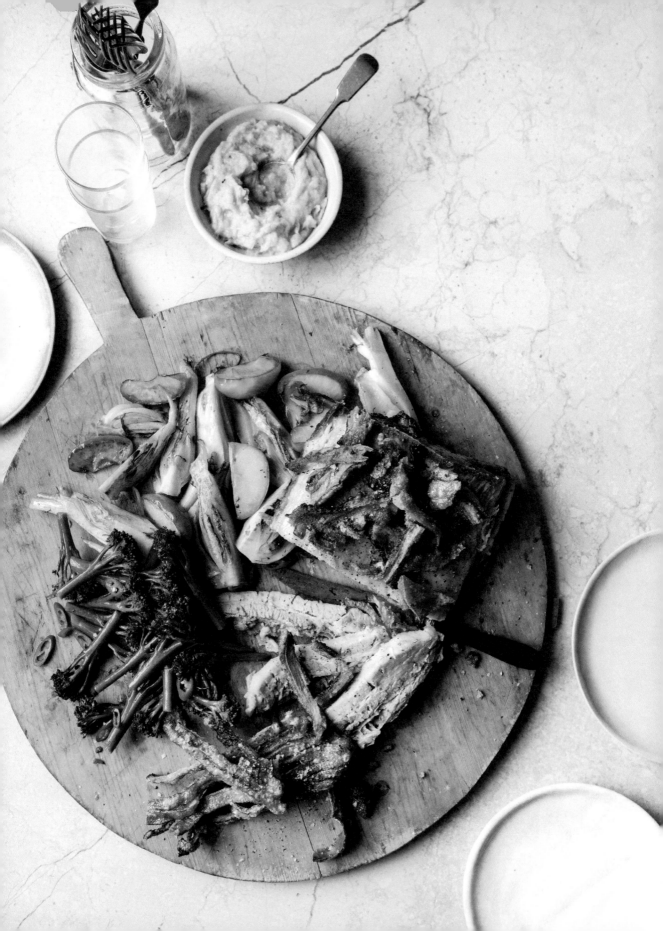

Ginger beef and cavolo nero

This is a lovely perky dish that can work perfectly on its own or with some rice noodles or quinoa.

Serves: 2

olive oil, for cooking
2 cloves garlic, finely chopped
5cm (2 inches) root ginger, peeled
  and cut into fine matchsticks
1 sirloin steak, sliced into thin strips
5–6 long cavolo nero leaves, finely
  shredded
2 teaspoons light soy sauce
1 teaspoon honey
¼ teaspoon Chinese five-spice powder
sea salt

Heat a little oil in a wok or wide pan. Throw in the garlic and ginger, along with a pinch of salt, and stir-fry for 2–3 minutes.

Add the strips of steak and continue to stir-fry for 3–4 minutes. Add the cavolo nero and stir-fry for 1 minute more.

Add the soy sauce, honey and five-spice powder and stir-fry for another 2 minutes, until the honey caramelizes and turns a little sticky.

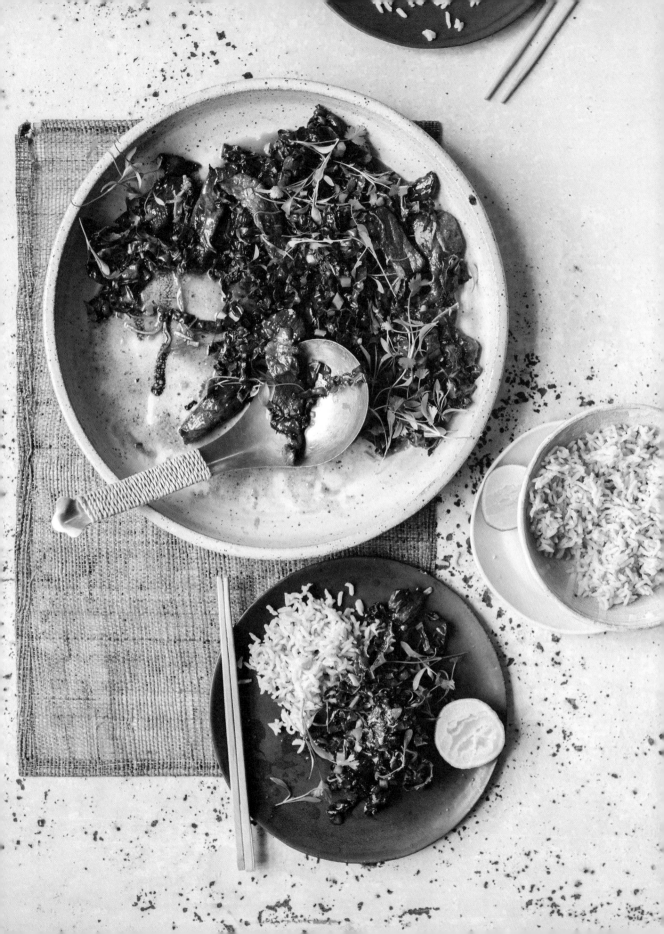

Venison sausage and rosemary stew with sweet potato mash

This makes an incredibly nutrient-dense, filling and low-GI family dinner.

Serves: 4–5

olive oil, for cooking and drizzling
2 red onions, finely sliced
2 cloves garlic, finely chopped
6 slices streaky bacon, cut into small pieces
2 star anise
12 venison sausages
3 bay leaves
2 large sprigs rosemary

1 teaspoon smoked paprika
1 x 400g (14oz) can chopped tomatoes
200ml (generous ¾ cup) chicken stock
1 tablespoon light soy sauce
100ml (scant ½ cup) red wine
1 x 400g (14oz) can chickpeas (garbanzo beans), drained
2 large sweet potatoes, peeled and diced
sea salt and black pepper

Preheat the oven to 180°C/350°F/Gas mark 4.

Heat a little olive oil in a large frying pan, add the onions, garlic, bacon, star anise and a pinch of salt and sauté until the onion is beginning to soften. Prick the sausages, add to the pan and continue to sauté until the sausages start to brown. Transfer everything to a casserole dish and stir in the bay leaves, rosemary, paprika, tomatoes, stock, soy sauce, red wine and chickpeas (garbanzo beans).

Place the lid on the dish and bake for 40–50 minutes, checking occasionally; you want the liquid to have reduced to a thick sauce and the flavours to have intensified.

While the casserole is cooking, boil the diced sweet potato until soft. Drain, then add a small drizzle of olive oil and some salt and pepper, and mash well.

Serve the casserole with a generous dollop of mash.

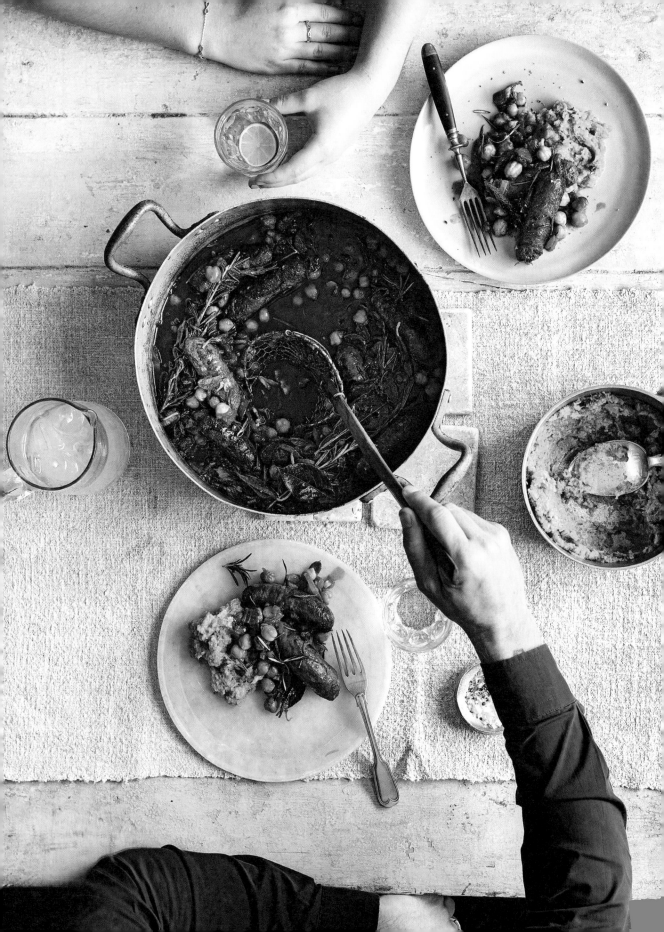

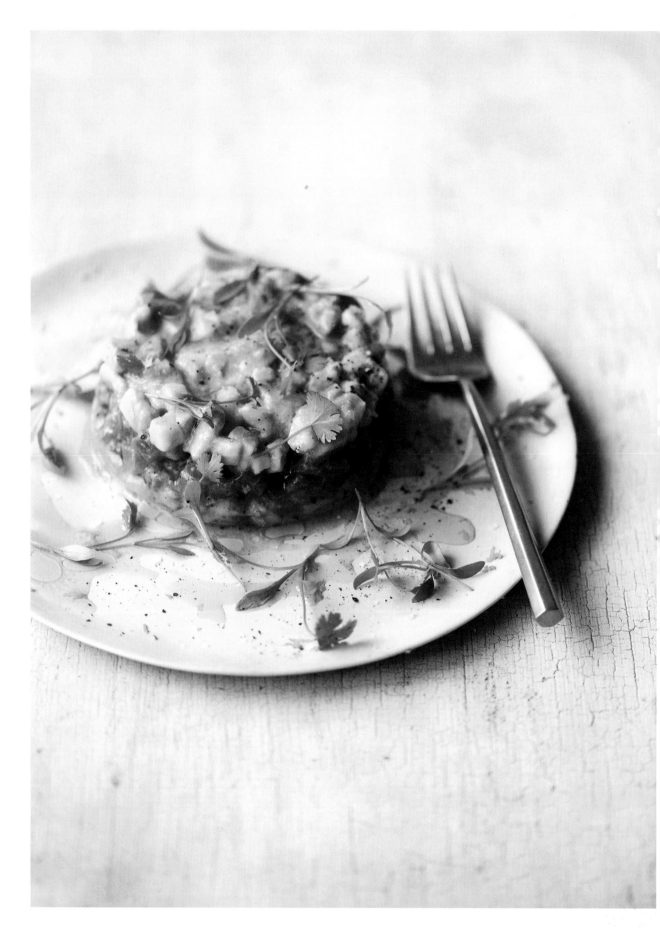

Tuna carpaccio with orange dressing

This is a great little starter. A note of caution, though: check with your fishmonger that the tuna is very fresh. If in ANY doubt, leave it out!

Serves: 1

1 ripe avocado
6 tablespoons extra virgin olive oil
1 extremely fresh tuna steak
juice of ½ orange
sea salt and black pepper

Roughly dice the avocado flesh and put into a small bowl. Add 2 tablespoons of the oil with salt and pepper to taste, and mix well with a fork, which will produce a creamier texture.

Very finely slice the tuna, then cut into small dice.

Put the orange juice and the remaining oil in a small bowl, with salt and pepper to taste, and whisk well. Add the diced tuna to the orange dressing and stir gently to coat.

Place a 10-cm (4-inch) round metal pastry cutter on a plate and spoon one-quarter of the avocado mixture into the bottom, pushing it down to create the first layer. Then use a fork to remove the diced tuna from the dressing, allowing the excess dressing to drip back into the bowl, and place the tuna dice on top of the avocado layer. Top with another quarter of the avocado. Push down firmly then gently pull the pastry cutter away to reveal a round, 3-tiered dish. Repeat with the rest of the ingredients on a second plate.

Feel-good fish fingers

Who said fish fingers had to be junk food? This simple version creates a fish finger that is rich in omega-3 fatty acids and is junk-free. Awesome!

Serves: 2

2 tablespoons ground flaxseed
2 tablespoons fine oatmeal
½ teaspoon garlic granules
½ teaspoon dried mixed herbs
2 large, skinless salmon fillets
olive oil, for coating
sea salt and black pepper
lemon wedges, to serve

Preheat the oven to 200°C/400°F/Gas mark 6.

Mix the ground flaxseed, oatmeal, garlic granules and dried herbs together, with salt and pepper to taste. Spread this mixture out on a flat surface.

Cut the salmon into fingers and lightly coat in olive oil. Roll the fingers in the flaxseed and oatmeal mixture until they are completely covered. Place on a baking sheet and bake in the oven for around 25 minutes, or until the coating is crisp and golden. Serve with lemon wedges.

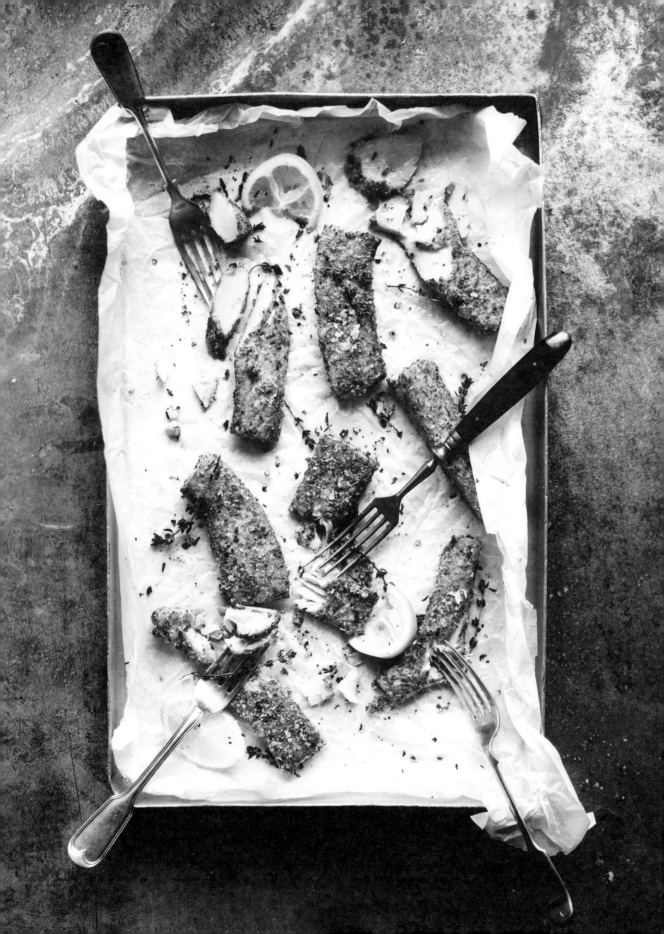

Snappy citrus tuna

This is a super-quick way to get a tasty lunch or dinner together. Citrus matches tuna steak beautifully. This can be served with a green salad, cooked vegetables, stir-fried noodles, brown rice – whatever takes your fancy.

Serves: 1

finely grated zest of 1 lime and juice of ½
1 teaspoon light soy sauce
1 teaspoon toasted sesame oil
2 teaspoons olive oil
1 tuna steak

Mix the lime zest and juice, soy sauce and oils together in a bowl and whisk well.

Place the tuna in the liquid and rotate it a few times to ensure it is well covered.

Heat a frying pan or griddle pan until hot, remove the tuna from the liquid and cook for 3 minutes on each side, drizzling small amounts of the liquid over the tuna constantly as it cooks (this helps to get the flavours into the fish and also gives it some colour).

Cut the tuna into slices to serve.

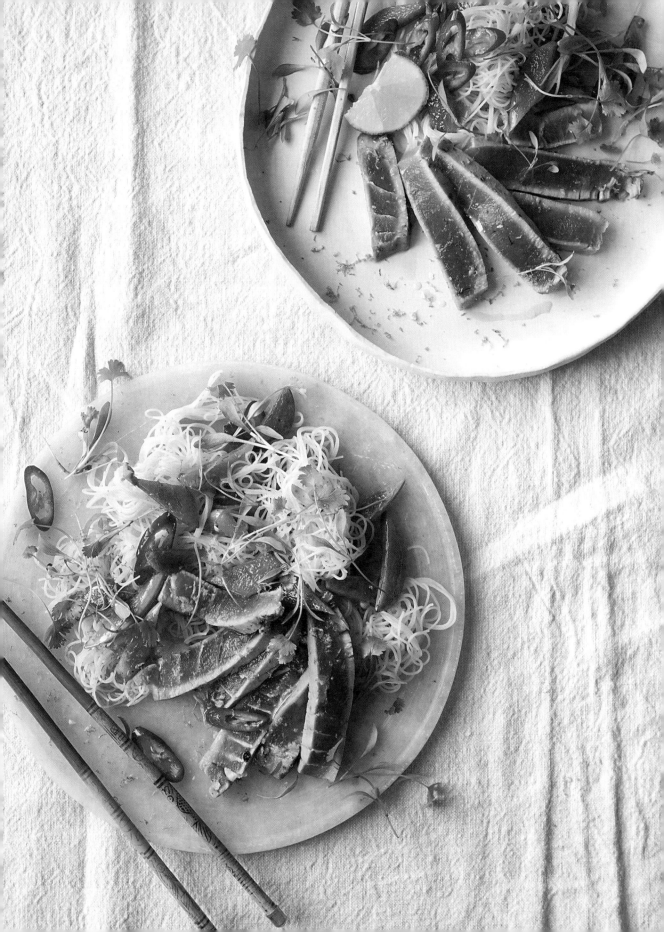

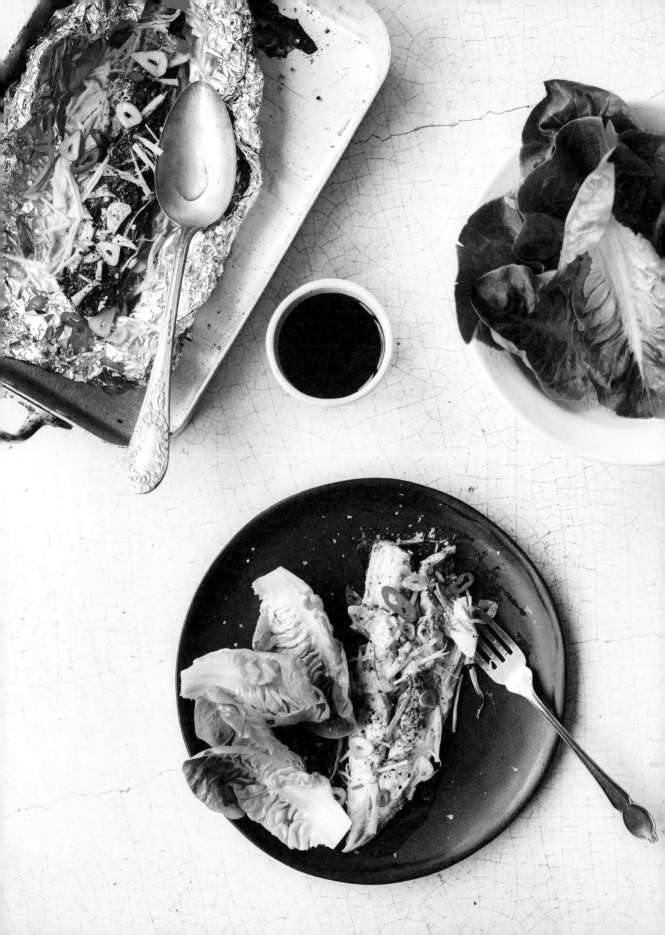

Asian-style mackerel foil parcels

These parcels are a speedy and fuss-free way of preparing tasty fish dishes, and a great way to capture lots of flavour. There really is no limit to the flavourings you can throw in the parcels.

Serves: 2

2 mackerel fillets
2.5cm (1 inch) root ginger, peeled
 and cut into matchsticks
2 cloves garlic, sliced
1 small red chilli (chile), sliced
juice of ½ lime
sea salt and black pepper

Preheat the oven to 180°C/350°F/Gas mark 4. Place 2 sheets of foil on a work surface and bunch each up into a bowl shape.

Place a mackerel fillet in each foil bowl. Sprinkle half the ginger, garlic and chilli (chile) over each mackerel fillet. Squeeze over the lime juice and season with salt and pepper. Scrunch the top of each parcel together to enclose and seal.

Place on a roasting tray and bake in the oven 25 minutes. Serve with a green salad.

Salmon curry

I absolutely adore salmon in a curry. It may seem slightly unconventional, but it has been becoming more and more popular in recent years. It's a perfect way to get those important omega-3 fatty acids in.

Serves: 2

olive oil, for cooking
1 red onion, finely chopped
3 cloves garlic, finely chopped
1 whole small red chilli (chile), finely chopped
2 star anise
1 cinnamon stick

200g (heaped 1 cup) red lentils
1–2 tablespoons mild curry paste
400ml (1¾ cups) coconut milk
1 sweet potato, diced (skin left on)
about 500ml (generous 2 cups) vegetable stock
2 skinless salmon fillets, cut into large dice

Heat a little oil in a pan and sauté the onion, garlic, chilli (chile), star anise and cinnamon until the onion starts to soften.

Add the lentils, curry paste and coconut milk, stir well and simmer for a few minutes. Add the sweet potato and, after a few minutes, start adding the stock a little at a time. Continue simmering for around 15–20 minutes, stirring frequently and adding more stock if necessary, to give the dish a porridge-like consistency.

Add the salmon and continue to simmer for another 4–5 minutes, stirring very lightly so as not to break it up, until the salmon is just cooked. Remove the cinnamon sticks and star anise before serving.

Salmon with avocado and dill yogurt sauce

This is a great sauce to go with salmon. It works well with freshly cooked salmon, but also smoked salmon and poached eggs. Pretty versatile really.

Serves: 2

2 salmon fillets

For the sauce
1 very large avocado
2 tablespoons Greek yogurt
3 tablespoons chopped dill
1 clove garlic, finely chopped
juice of 1 lemon
sea salt and black pepper

Preheat the oven to 180°C/350°F/Gas mark 4.

Bake the salmon in the oven for around 20 minutes.

To make the sauce, place all the ingredients in a food processor and blitz into a smooth sauce. Serve with the salmon.

Miso salmon with garlic spinach and carrot ginger purée

This is such a gorgeous dish: a combination of a few of my favourites from around the world. It is pretty simple, but has a rich, complex flavour and is a great one to pull out of the bag at dinner parties. White miso is available online and in many supermarkets. It is important not to use brown miso here, as it is too salty.

Serves: 2

3 large carrots, cut into chunks
1.25cm (½ inch) root ginger, peeled
  and finely chopped
about 400ml (1¾ cups) vegetable stock
1 tablespoon sweet white miso
2 teaspoons toasted sesame oil

1 teaspoon honey
olive oil, for oiling and cooking
2 salmon fillets
1 clove garlic, finely chopped
2 large handfuls baby spinach
sea salt

Preheat the oven to 180°C/350°F/Gas mark 4.

Place the carrots and ginger in a saucepan and add enough stock to almost cover the carrots. Simmer until the carrots are soft, then blend to a smooth purée; keep warm.

Mix the miso, sesame oil and honey with 2 teaspoons water.

Lightly oil a baking sheet and lay the salmon fillets on the sheet. Spread the miso mixture over the salmon, reserving some. Bake at the top of the oven for 25 minutes, spreading the remaining miso mixture over the salmon halfway through cooking.

Sauté the garlic in a little olive oil, with a pinch of salt, for about 2 minutes until it begins to turn aromatic. Add the spinach and sauté until wilted.

To serve, add a generous spoonful of carrot ginger purée to 2 plates and spread it out. Place the spinach on top, then add the salmon fillets.

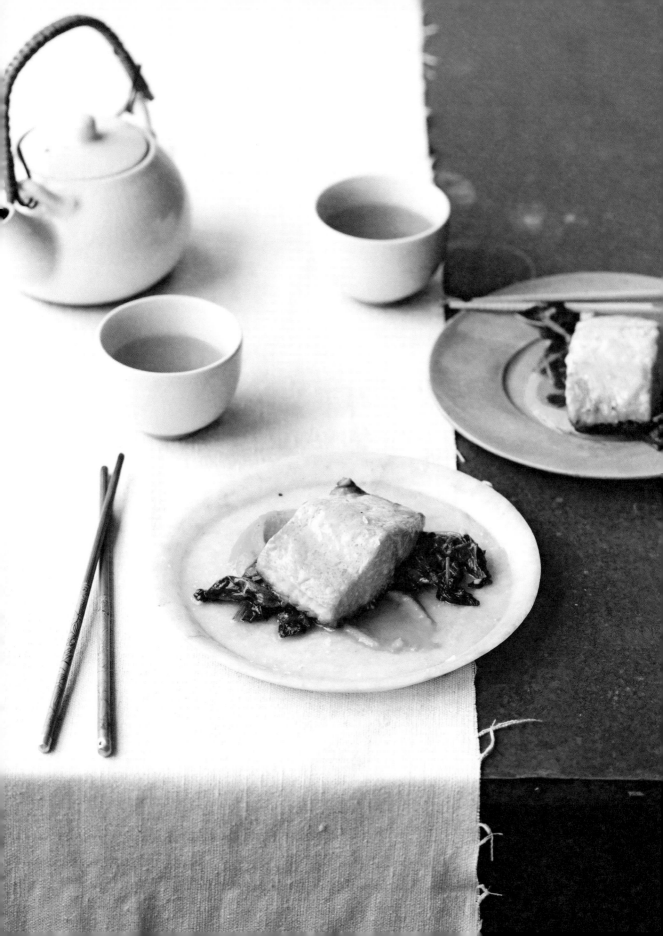

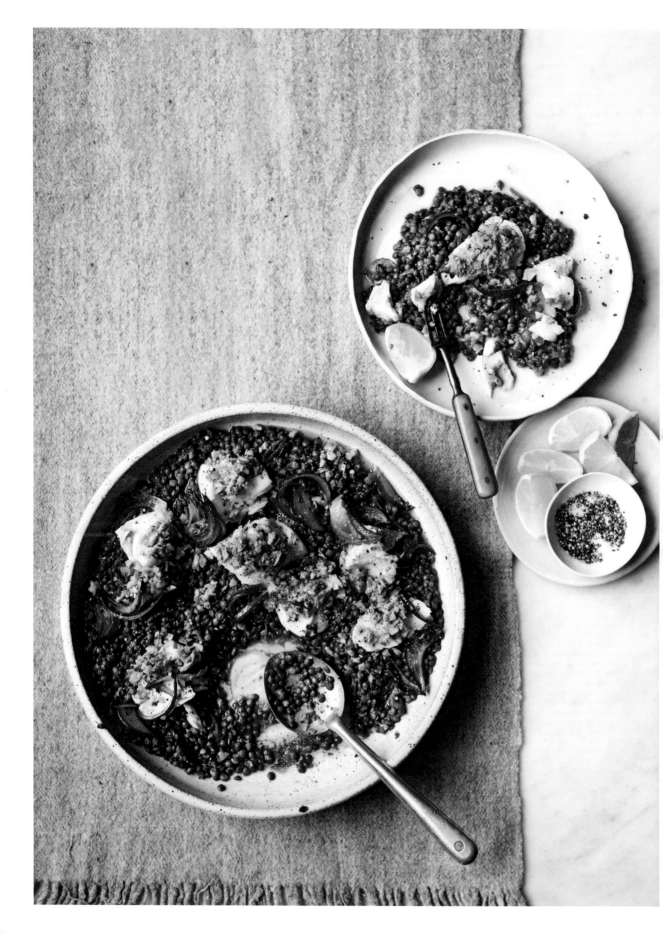

Cod with green olive tapenade and Puy lentils

This dish is serious – loads of flavour, filling and comforting! Tapenade is easy to make, but it is readily available in supermarkets too, so for ease I have opted for that here.

Serves: 2

olive oil, for cooking and oiling
1 red onion, finely chopped
2 cloves garlic, finely chopped
250g (1⅓ cups) Puy lentils
about 500ml (generous 2 cups)
   vegetable stock
¼ teaspoon cornflour (cornstarch)
2 cod fillets
2 tablespoons green olive tapenade
lemon wedges, to serve

Preheat the oven to 180°C/350°F/Gas mark 4.

Heat a little olive oil in a pan, add the onion and garlic and sauté until the onion begins to soften. Add the Puy lentils and a small amount of vegetable stock and allow to simmer. As the liquid reduces, add a little more stock, continuing in this way until the lentils are tender (Puy lentils don't break down in the same way as red lentils).

Mix the cornflour (cornstarch) with a small amount of water, then stir into the lentils. This will thicken the sauce in a few seconds. Set aside and keep warm.

Lightly oil a baking sheet and place the cod fillets on the sheet. Bake in the oven for 10 minutes, then spread the tapenade over the fillets and bake for another 10–15 minutes.

Serve the lentils and cod with lemon wedges.

Sesame-crusted tuna with lime, mango and chilli coulis and wilted pak choi

This looks a lot more demanding to make than it actually is. Just try to buy the freshest tuna possible.

Serves: 2

olive oil, for cooking
225g (8oz) pak choi (bok choy)
3 tablespoons sesame seeds
2 tuna steaks
sea salt and black pepper

For the coulis
1 large, very ripe mango, peeled, pitted and roughly chopped
juice of ½ lime
¼ red onion, roughly chopped
1 small red chilli (chile)

Begin by making the coulis. Place the mango, lime juice, red onion and chilli (chile) in a blender and blend to a smooth purée. Pour this mixture through a fine sieve into a saucepan, pushing it through with a spoon.

Heat a little oil in a frying pan and gently sauté the pak choi (bok choy) until wilted.

Sprinkle the sesame seeds onto a large plate and mix in a little salt and pepper. Lay the tuna steaks on the sesame seeds and press down so that the seeds stick. Flip the tuna and coat the other sides in the same way.

Heat 1 tablespoon oil in a wide frying pan and, when hot, gently place the sesame-coated tuna in the pan. Fry for about 3 minutes on each side, turning them as gently as possible so as not to knock the seeds off.

Warm through the coulis and the pak choi. Divide the pak choi between 2 plates, placing it in the centre. Slice the tuna steak and place it on top of the pak choi, then drizzle the coulis over the top.

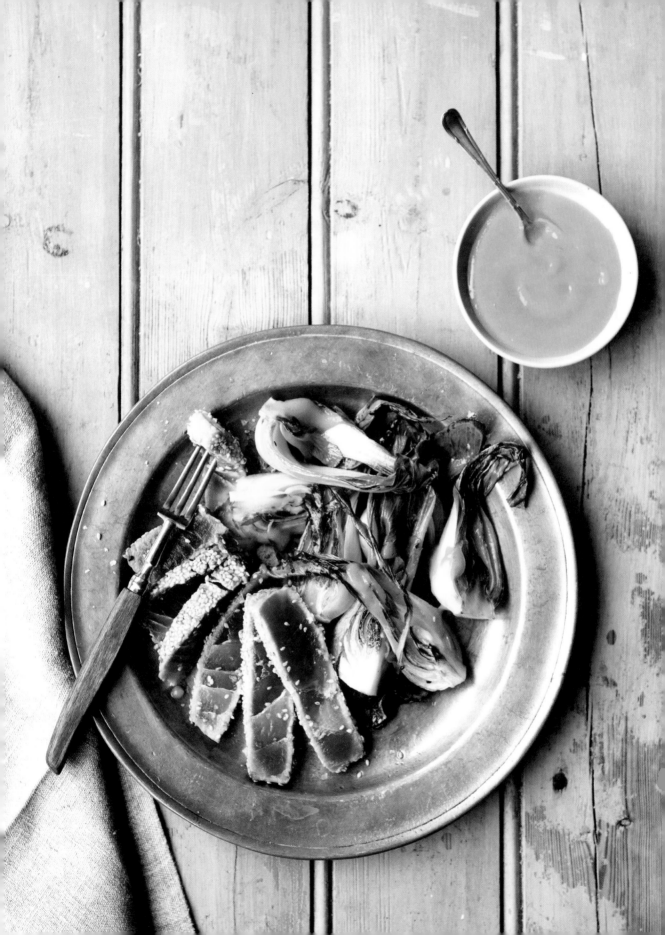

Sea bass with smashed pea and feta crust and garlic cavolo nero

This is a lovely, fresh, tasty dish. Super-simple with plenty of flavour.

Serves: 2

4 tablespoons frozen garden peas
2 slices feta cheese
olive oil, for oiling and cooking
2 sea bass fillets
2 cloves garlic, finely chopped
6 long cavolo nero leaves, shredded
sea salt and black pepper

Preheat the oven to 180°C/350°F/Gas mark 4.

Place the peas in a small saucepan and cover with boiling water. Simmer for 6–8 minutes then drain and crush the peas with a fork. Crumble the feta cheese into the crushed peas along with a pinch of black pepper, and mix well.

Lightly oil a baking sheet. Lay the sea bass fillets on the baking sheet. Spoon the pea mixture over the fillets and bake in the oven for around 20 minutes.

Meanwhile, heat a little olive oil and sauté the garlic with a pinch of salt for about 2 minutes. Throw in the shredded cavolo nero and sauté until it turns a deep green and softens.

Serve the sea bass with the garlic cavolo nero.

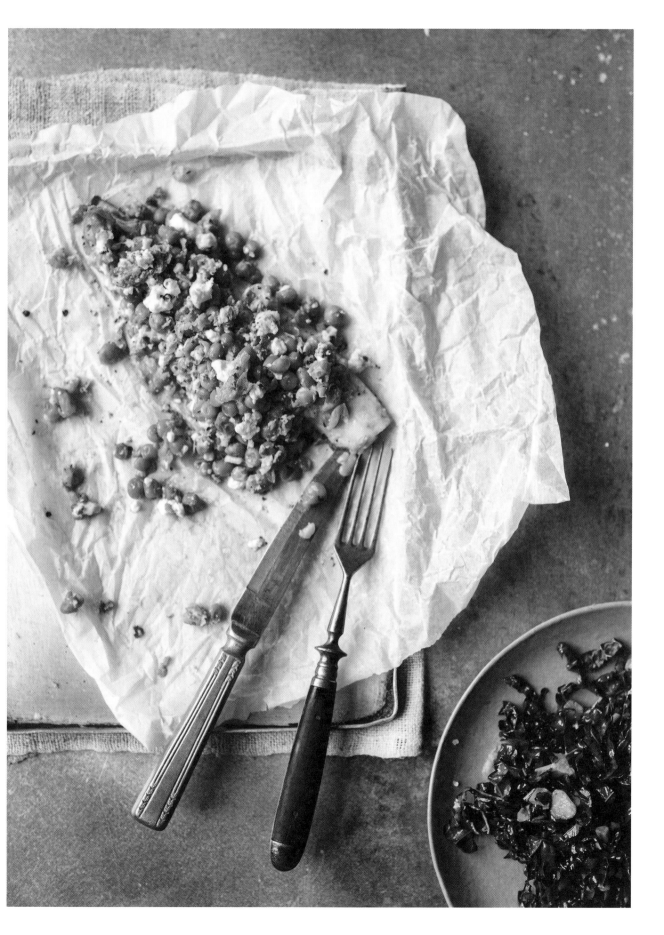

Citrus ginger salmon parcels

Small paper parcels are a great way to combine lots of flavours together in a small, compact little unit. All manner of herbs and spices can be added to these, so get creative and experiment with as many different options as you can.

Serves: 1

1 salmon fillet
2.5cm (1 inch) root ginger, peeled
    and cut into thin matchsticks
½ red chilli (chile), finely chopped
2 slices lemon
sea salt and cracked black pepper

Shape a piece of baking parchment into a bowl or open-topped parcel; it doesn't have to be pretty, as long as it contains all the ingredients and the top remains open.

Lay the salmon fillet inside the parchment bowl. Sprinkle some salt and pepper over the fillet, then sprinkle the ginger and chilli (chile) over, and finally top with the lemon slices.

Steam for 15 minutes.

Prawns with spring onions, ginger and lemon

This is a lovely fresh dish that works well with some cooked quinoa and greens, or even as a snack on its own.

Serves: 1–2

1 tablespoon olive oil
2 cloves garlic, finely chopped
2.5cm (1 inch) root ginger, peeled and
   cut into matchsticks
4 spring onions (scallions), halved
   across the middle, then sliced
   lengthways into strips
115g (4oz) cooked king prawns (shrimp)
1 teaspoon honey
juice of ½ lemon

Heat the oil in a wok or wide pan. Throw in the garlic, ginger and spring onions (scallions) and stir-fry for around 3–4 minutes.

Add the prawns (shrimp), honey and lemon juice and simmer for a minute or so before serving.

Spiced griddled squid

I'm absolutely obsessed with squid. It is incredibly high in that all-important selenium, alongside good amounts of zinc, which supports immune health. This is great served in a salad, with a few rocket (arugula) leaves as a starter, or even with some cooked quinoa.

Serves: 1

olive oil, for oiling
2–3 prepared squid tubes

For the spice mix
¼ teaspoon ground cinnamon
¼ teaspoon smoked paprika
¼ teaspoon ground cumin
¼ teaspoon garlic granules
sea salt and black pepper

Mix the spices together in a small bowl, with salt and pepper to taste.

Lightly oil a griddle pan and place over a high heat until hot.

Sprinkle a good coating of the spice mix onto each side of the squid tubes. Lay the squid gently in the hot pan and cook for 1–2 minutes, then turn and repeat on the other side before serving hot.

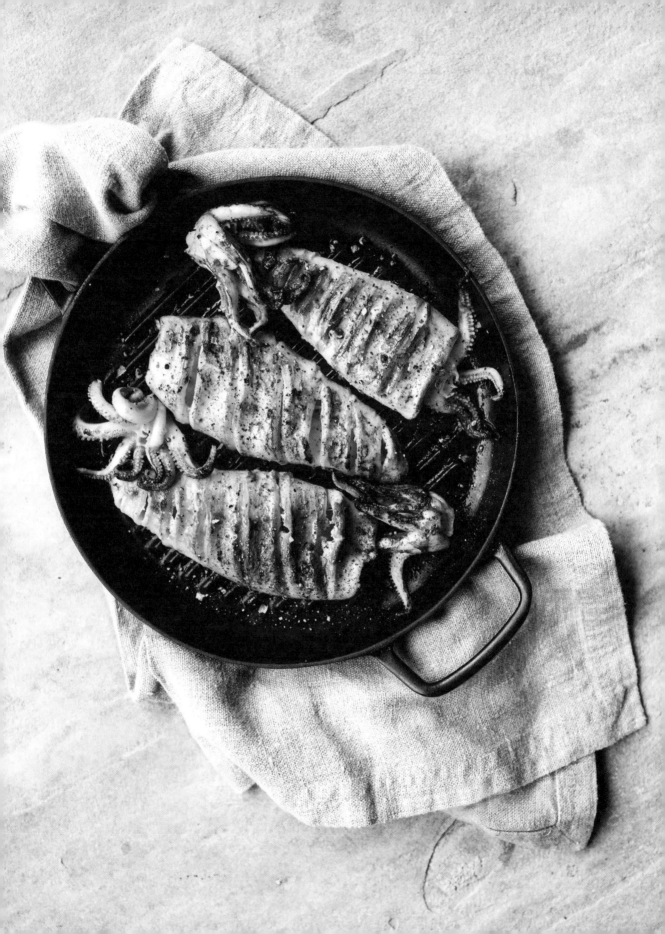

Scallops and chorizo with celeriac purée

I adore this combination, which is sweet, salty and earthy. I can't exactly pretend that chorizo is on the top of the healthy ingredients list, but this small amount adds a gorgeous flavour. By all means leave it out if you really want to.

Serves: 2

olive oil, for cooking
½ white onion, finely chopped
1 clove garlic, finely chopped
¼ large celeriac, peeled and diced
200–300ml (generous ¾–1¼ cups)
  vegetable stock
6 chunks eating chorizo
6 large scallops, white part only
sea salt and black pepper

Heat a little oil in a pan, add the onion, garlic and a good pinch of salt and sauté until the onion is soft. Add the celeriac and enough stock to almost cover the celeriac. Simmer until the celeriac is soft, then purée to a smooth, thick-soup consistency.

Pan-fry the chorizo slices (they won't need any oil) for 2 minutes until cooked and turning crisp at the edges.

Heat a clean frying pan with a little oil, add the scallops and pan-fry gently for 2–3 minutes on each side, until the edges begin to turn lovely and golden.

Place a layer of the celeriac purée on each plate. Add 3 slices of the chorizo on top of the purée. Top the chorizo slices with the scallops, season with black pepper and serve straight away.

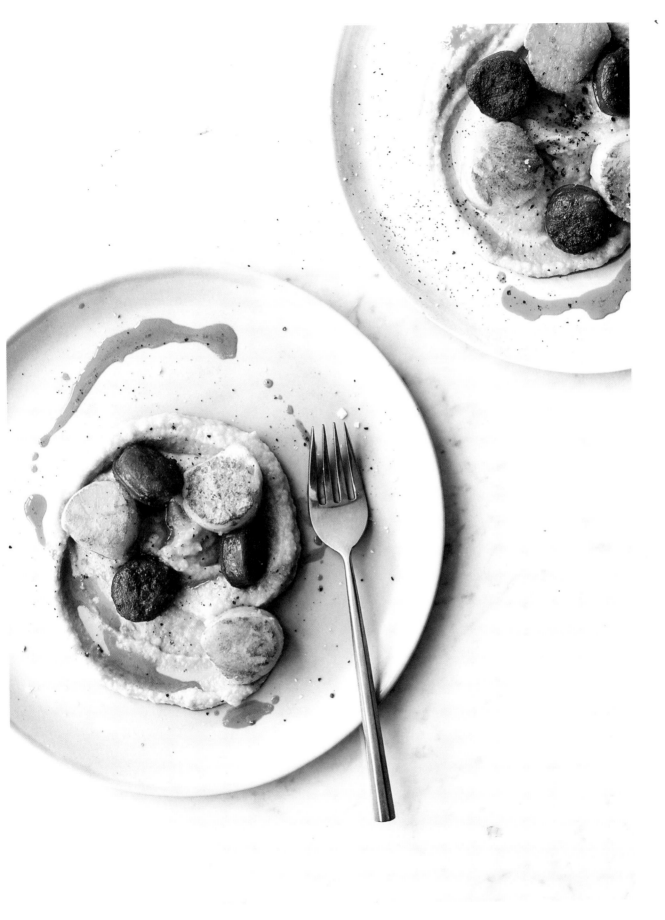

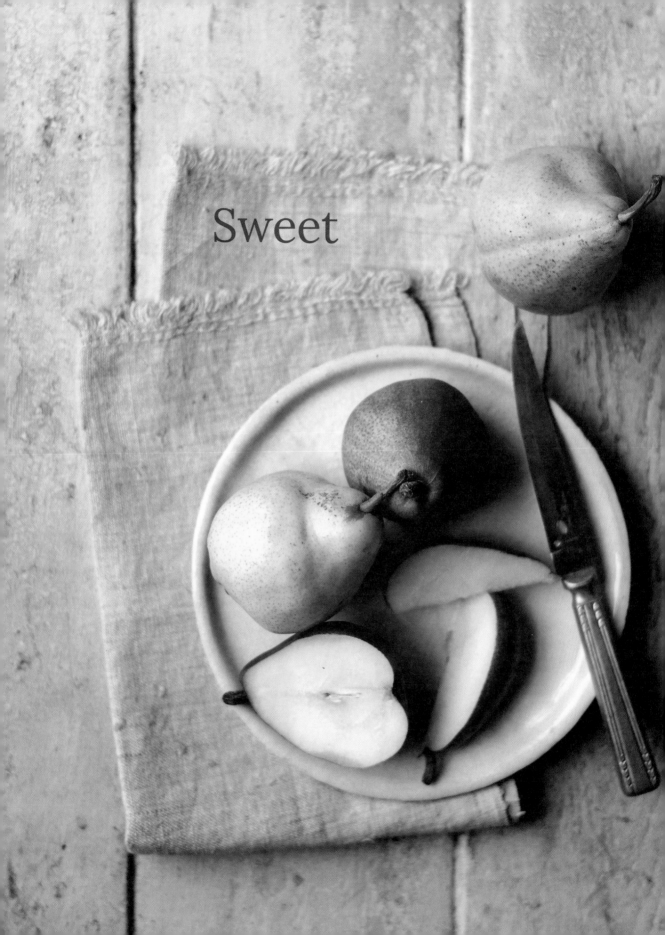

Sweet

Matcha bliss balls

Matcha is Japanese green tea powder. Its flavour is absolutely divine and it is packed up to the eyeballs with antioxidants.

Serves: 2

120g (4¼oz) dates
100g (3½oz) cashew nuts
65g (2¼oz) shelled pistachios
1 heaped tablespoon coconut oil
2 heaped teaspoons matcha powder
desiccated (dried shredded) coconut,
   for coating

Place all the ingredients except the desiccated (dried shredded) coconut in a food processor and pulse until a smooth, green, nutty dough has formed.

Break off thumb-sized pieces of the dough and roll into balls. Roll the balls through the coconut to coat, then place on a plate and refrigerate for a few hours to set.

See photograph on page 174.

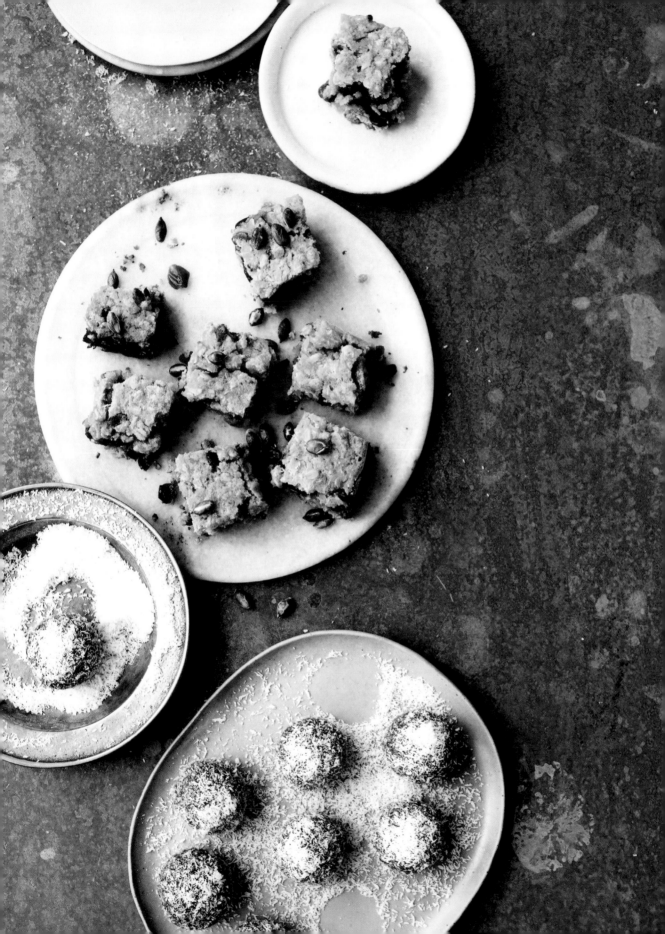

Mini coconut cake bites

These great little cake bites are perfect when you want something that tastes naughty, looks naughty, but won't destroy your attempts to eat better. Coconut flour is a very filling, very low-glycaemic alternative to regular flour.

Serves: 3–4

75g (2½oz) coconut flour
175g (scant 2 cups) porridge oats
2 tablespoons pumpkin seeds
2 tablespoons dried cranberries
finely grated zest and juice of
   1 large orange
100g (3½oz) coconut oil, melted
4 tablespoons honey
4 eggs
1 jar of mincemeat (or mixed dried fruit)

Preheat the oven to 200°C/400°F/Gas mark 6.

Combine the coconut flour, oats, pumpkin seeds, dried cranberries and orange zest in a bowl and mix thoroughly. Add the melted coconut oil and honey and stir to mix. Add the orange juice and stir.

Crack the eggs into the mixture one at a time, mixing well between each addition. When a firm, doughy cake mix has formed, spread half of it into the base of a small greased cake tin.

Spoon the mincemeat over the mixture and spread it out evenly. Add the remaining cake mixture on top and bake in the oven for 15–20 minutes, until golden. Leave to cool completely before cutting into small squares.

Chilli chocolate Brazils

These are a great little snack to have on hand in the fridge when you feel the need for a chocolate fix. They are actually very nutrient-dense: the Brazil nuts are packed with selenium and the chocolate is rich in heart-healthy flavonoids. Bargain!

Serves: 3–4

300g (10½oz) dark chocolate (80% cocoa solids), broken into pieces
pinch cayenne pepper
30 Brazil nuts

Quarter-fill a saucepan with boiling water (off the heat) and place a glass heatproof bowl over the pan so the base is not touching the hot water. Add the chocolate to the bowl with the cayenne pepper, then stir continuously until all the chocolate has melted.

Add a few Brazil nuts at a time to the melted chocolate to coat, then fish them out with a fork and place them straight onto a baking sheet lined with baking parchment. Transfer to the fridge for about 30 minutes, for the chocolate to set.

● SWEETS AND SNACKS
● GOOD FATS
✗ PERFECT FOR DESSERT

Raw pot au chocolat

I am a big fan of "pot au chocolat", and this is a much healthier version that uses avocado as the base, giving the same mouthfeel as a rich chocolate dessert but without all the junk. (Avocados can also be used to make chocolate mousse.) Adding coconut oil helps it set a little to give the dessert the texture of a smooth chocolate ganache.

Serves: 2

1 large, very ripe avocado
4 tablespoons cocoa powder
1 tablespoon honey
1 heaped tablespoon coconut oil, melted

Scoop the avocado flesh into a food processor.

Add the cocoa powder, honey and melted coconut oil and blitz until smooth. Taste it at this point (natural variation in avocados can affect the flavour) and add more honey if you feel it needs to be sweeter or more cocoa if it needs to be richer. Blitz again, transfer to small pots and chill in the fridge for a few hours.

Black and blue parfaits

This is a super-speedy dessert that can be thrown together easily and provides you with plenty of antioxidants. The berries and a spoonful of honey should provide sufficient sweetness.

Serves: 2

75g (2½oz) blueberries
75g (2½oz) blackberries
8 tablespoons plain yogurt
2 teaspoons honey

Spoon a layer of berries into 2 tall glasses, then a layer of yogurt, then berries, then yogurt, and so on until you reach the top of the glass.

Drizzle a teaspoon of honey over the top of each and serve.

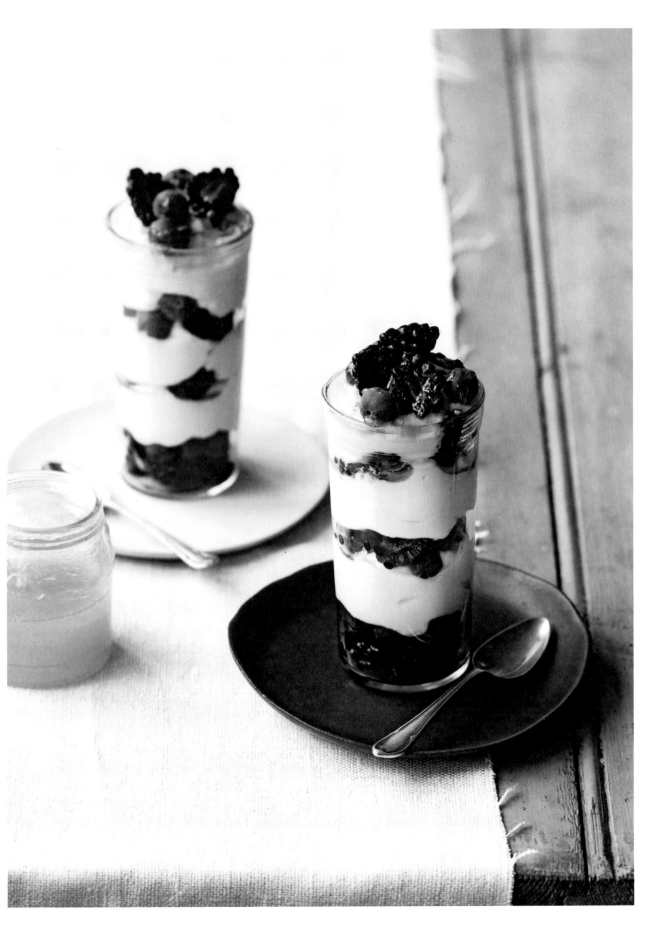

Crunchy fruit crumble

I do love a good crumble; for me, it has "family Sunday lunch" written all over it! While traditionally it would contain loads of sugar, it really doesn't need to – a good selection of fruit will give it enough sweetness.

Serves: 2–3

75g (2½oz) blueberries
75g (2½oz) blackberries
1 ripe mango, diced
1 apple, cored and diced
1 cinnamon stick
1 star anise
about 50g (½ cup) porridge oats

Preheat the oven to 200°C/400°F/Gas mark 6.

Place all the fruit and spices in a saucepan over a high heat and simmer until the fruits are starting to break down.

Transfer to an ovenproof dish and sprinkle over enough oats to completely cover the fruit. Bake in the oven for 20 minutes, or until the oats start to turn golden brown and crunchy.

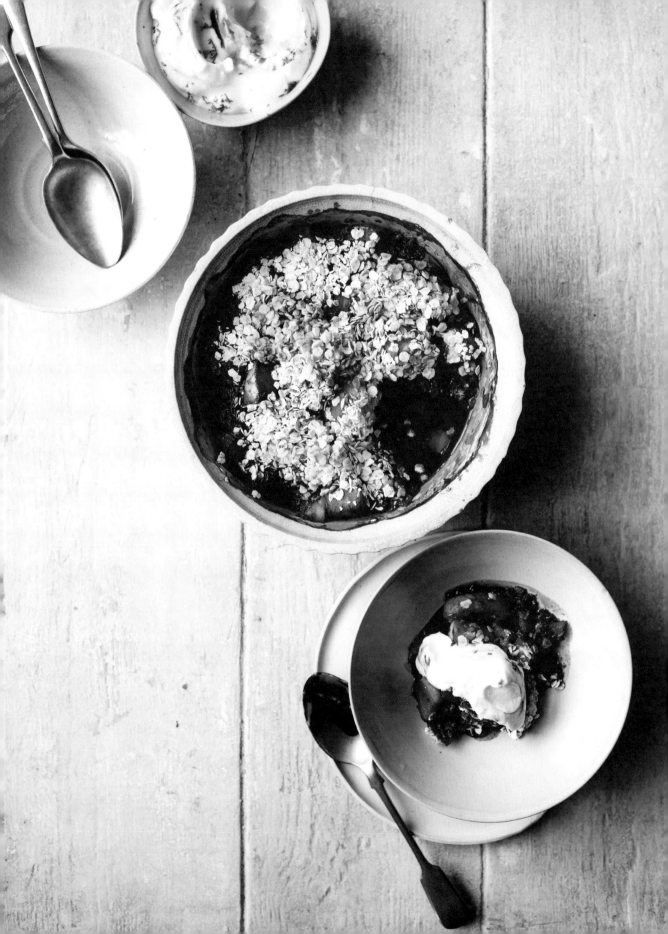

● SWEETS AND SNACKS
○ WHOLE GRAINS
✗ PERFECT FOR DESSERT

Goji berry cheesecake

Although this is called a cheesecake, the filling is actually tofu (bean curd). Now, before you get worried, it's not going to be bland slop – the tofu here is just texture and a flavour carrier, but with a lot fewer calories than a traditional cheesecake.

Serves: 4

For the base
250g (12½oz) oatcakes, crushed
125g (generous ¾ cup) butter, melted

For the goji berry sauce
300g (10½oz) goji berries
juice of ½ lemon, plus zest to decorate

For the filling
400g (14oz) firm tofu (bean curd)
1 teaspoon cornflour (cornstarch)
2 tablespoons honey
1 tablespoon coconut oil, melted

Begin by making the base. Combine the crushed oatcakes and melted butter well. Press the mixture into the base of a 20-cm/8-inch tart tin. Place in the fridge.

To prepare the sauce, place the goji berries in a bowl, add enough cold water to cover them and set aside to soak.

For the filling, put the tofu (bean curd), cornflour (cornstarch), honey and melted coconut oil into a food processor and process to a smooth, creamy filling.

Remove the chilled base from the fridge and pour the filling over the base. Tap the tin gently on the work surface to ensure that the filling is evenly spread. Return to the fridge for 4 hours.

Ten minutes before serving, strain the goji berries, reserving the soaking water. Transfer the berries, lemon juice and 2 tablespoons of the soaking water to a food processor and blitz to a sauce – it will have a little texture and some seeds in it.

Decorate the cheesecake with lemon zest and serve with the sauce.

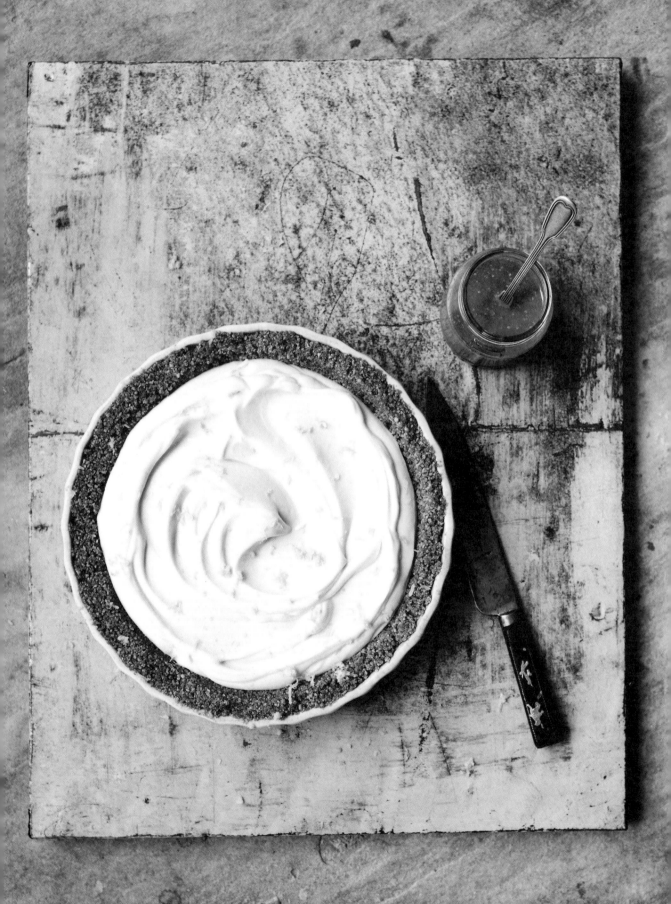

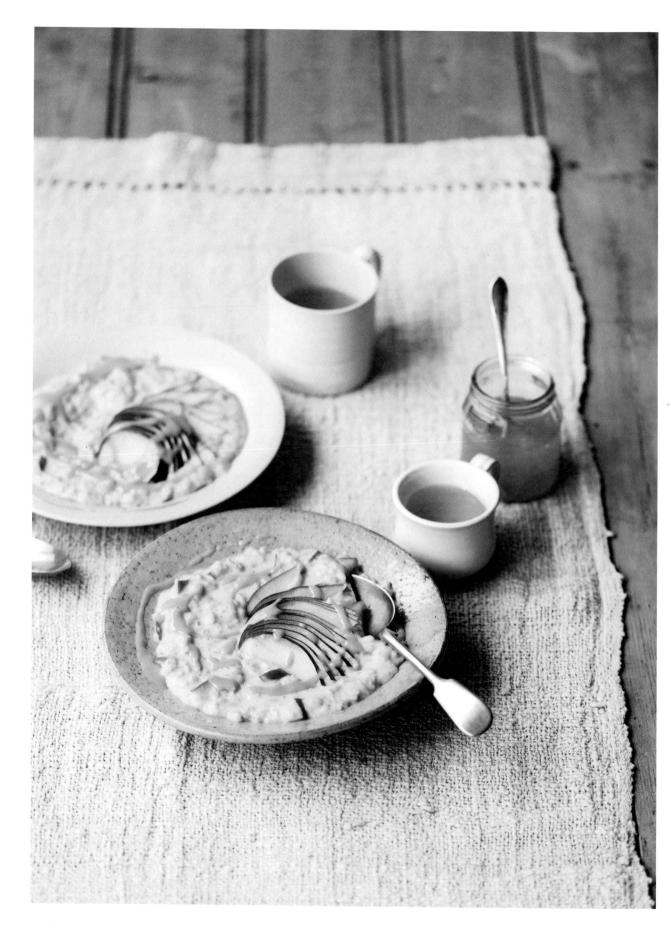

● SWEETS AND SNACKS
● WHOLE GRAINS
✗ PERFECT FOR BREAKFAST

Pear and tahini porridge

This is a gorgeous, indulgent breakfast that has several levels of flavour, not to mention a rich diversity of nutrients.

Serves: 2

1 tablespoon tahini
½ teaspoon vanilla extract
1 pear
50g (½ cup) porridge oats
350ml (1½ cups) milk (regular,
   or a dairy-free alternative)
1 teaspoon honey

Mix the tahini and vanilla extract together.

Cut the pear in half lengthways. Dice one half and cut the other half lengthways into slices.

Place the oats, milk, honey and diced pear in a pan and simmer for 4–5 minutes, then transfer to 2 bowls. Fan the pear slices on top of the porridge and drizzle over the vanilla tahini to serve.

Index

Want to work in food, health, and wellness? Want to study without rigid time commitments and without breaking the bank?

Consider studying at Dale Pinnock's
THE SANO SCHOOL OF CULINARY MEDICINE

- Evidence based, applied, and practical.
- Study anywhere, anytime. Fit the course around your life.
- No tight deadlines or timescales, take as long as you want.
- Encourages *your* creativity and teaches you how to build recipes around the science with confidence.
- Developed by one of the country's leading voices in nutrition and health.

Accredited and CPD registered. Our 'Diploma in Culinary Medicine' has been accredited by the CMA and the FNTP, and has been awarded a value of 5 CPD points to qualified NTs by the FNTP

www.sanoschoolofculinarymedicine.com

Resources

DIABETES UK
The most widely known diabetes organization in the UK, their website is a great resource for information on diabetes and its management.
diabetes.org.uk

BRITISH HEART FOUNDATION
Probably the best known organization championing heart health, their website is a great resource for everything from statistics and medical breakthrough information, through to practical everyday tips for looking after your heart.
bhf.org.uk

BRITISH DIETETIC ASSOCIATION
Their factsheets are available for free. They comprise information about specific illnesses/disorders system health and also offer advice on dietary changes etc.
bda.uk.com/foodfacts/hypertension

CHRIS KRESSER
One of the top 25 natural health sites in the world.
chriskresser.com

MARK'S DAILY APPLE
Empowering people to take responsibility for their own health and enjoyment of life by investigating what's reported about health and wellness.
marksdailyapple.com

Acknowledgments

Thanks to Clare Hulton, Zoie Wainwright, and Kruger Cowne
– a management trio that have changed the world for me!

Tanya Murkett – as always, helping me find my smile.

The absolute dream team – Issy Croker, Emily Ezekiel, and
Anna Barnett, this book is just stunning thanks to you amazing trio.

Céline, Sarah, and all the Quadrille crew!

Doug, Heather, and all the team over at Sano – world domination, anyone?

Catherine Tyldesley, Gaby Roslin, Ramsay & Candy, Mum & Dad.

Publishing director: Sarah Lavelle
Creative director: Helen Lewis
Commissioning editor: Céline Hughes
Design concept: Nicola Ellis
Designer: Emily Lapworth
Photography: Issy Croker
Food and prop stylist: Emily Ezekiel
Food stylist's assistant: Anna Barnett
Production: Emily Noto, Vincent Smith

First published in 2017 by Quadrille Publishing
Pentagon House, 52–54 Southwark Street,
London SE1 1UN

Quadrille Publishing is an
imprint of Hardie Grant
www.hardiegrant.com.au
www.quadrille.co.uk

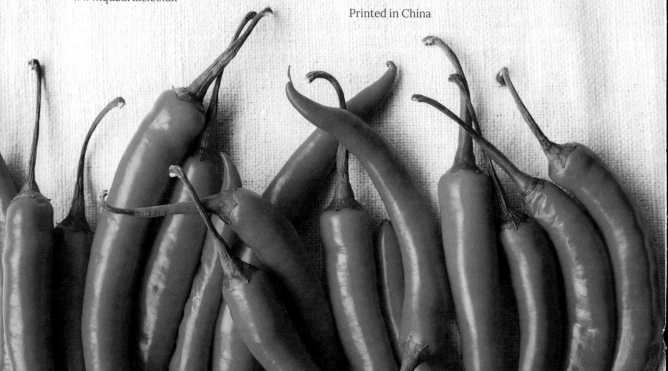